Foreword

One of the most promising ideas which has emerged from the recent reorganisation of the National Health Service is that Health Authorities should assess the needs of their populations, and then purchase and/or provide the services to meet them. Such an approach sets a new and stimulating agenda, with an explicit orientation towards the 'citizen-customer'.

Psychiatrists have worked in 'catchment areas' for many decades, and are thus more familiar with population-based planning than some other specialties. Interesting questions begin to arise: how and by whom are the needs, and their respective priorities, assessed? What is the evidence that a service is effective in meeting these needs? A key figure is, or should be, the Authority's Director of Public Health, planning, controlling and developing a needs-orientated service, by means of increasingly specific contracts. But how, and from whom does he or she get the necessary information?

It was these issues which set the agenda for the two conferences arranged by the Department of Health in Autumn 1990. It emerged that, in many Directors' reports, meeting the needs of the mentally ill hardly got a mention. Perhaps psychiatrists themselves are to blame for this state of affairs. At the meetings it was clear that there was a good deal of useful and sound data with which to make a start at addressing the questions. Conferences, while valuable, reach only a few. What is urgently required is an informed and active dialogue, at the level of every District, between local psychiatrists who have done their homework, and their Directors of Public Health. This publication points the way.

J L T Birley
25 January 1991

Past President of Royal College of Psychiatrists

Department of Health

Indicators for Mental Health in the Population

A Series of Two Workshops organised by the Faculty of Public Health Medicine, the Royal College of Psychiatrists and the Department of Health

◆

Workshop 1
Defining Needs
10 OCTOBER 1990

Workshop 2
Measuring Outcome
7 NOVEMBER 1990

Edited by Rachel Jenkins and Sian Griffiths

LONDON : HMSO

Hannibal House Department of Health Elephant and Castle London SE1

First published 1991

ISBN 0 11 321367 0

Contents

	Page
Acknowledgements	vii
List of Contributors	ix
Introduction	xi
Workshop 1: Defining Needs (*10 October 1990*)	
Introduction to Annual Reports of the Public Health *Dr Stephen Farrow*	1
Public Health and Psychiatric Morbidity *Professor Anthony Mann*	6
The Official Data Available on Mental Health *Dr Gyles Glover*	18
How can we measure Mental Health? *Dr Alastair Macdonald*	25
Filters to Care–A Model *Professor David Goldberg*	30
Applying a Model: Experiences from a District *Dr Alison Hill*	38
Contracting for Mental Health: What is Needed? *Dr Dinshaw Master and Claire Perry*	42
Discussion. Indicators for Need: their relevance to service provision	48
Workshop 2: Measuring Outcomes (*7 November 1990*)	
Setting Standards: A Service Blueprint *Professor Eugene Paykel*	50
Outcome Indicators of Mental Health *Dr Rachel Jenkins*	61
Audit in Mental Health *Professor John Wing*	87

Quality and Outcome Measurement in Mental Health Services: Community Care for Schizophrenic Patients in West Lambeth
Dr David Melzer 100

Implications for Public Health
Dr Sheila Adam 109

Discussion. Measurable Outcomes: their relevance to service provision 114

Acknowledgements

We are grateful to the Department of Health for sponsoring the workshops and providing the venue, to Rosemary McMahon of Professional Briefings for administration, to Lucy Sivoli and Dr Ruaridh Milne for their help in compiling the reports from the workshop discussion groups, and to the other group leaders and rapporteurs: Ann Farebrother, Andrew Stevens, Nicholas Salfield, Alastair Macdonald, Robin Murray, Neville Garratt, Michael Vaile, Sushma Acquilla, Deidre Cunningham, Rosemary Hunter, Graham Thornicroft, Terry Brugha and Adrian Lovett. Ian Wylie prepared the text for publication.

List of Contributors

Dr Jim Birley
Past President
Royal College of Psychiatrists

Dr Stephen Farrow
Director
Health Care Evaluation Unit
University of Bristol

Professor Anthony Mann
Professor of Epidemiological Psychiatry
Institute of Psychiatry

Dr Gyles Glover
Senior Lecturer in Community Medicine
Charing Cross and Westminster Medical School

Dr Alastair Macdonald
Consultant Psychogeriatrician and Senior Lecturer
Guy's Hospital

Professor David Goldberg
Department of Psychiatry
University of Manchester

Dr Alison Hill
Consultant in Public Health Medicine
Milton Keynes Health Authority

Dr Ruaridh Milne
Senior Registrar in Public Health Medicine
Oxford Regional Health Authority

Dr Dinshaw Master
Consultant Psychiatrist and Director of Mental Illness Services
Guy's Hospital

Ms Claire Perry
Director of Commissioning
Lewisham and North Southwark Health Authority

Dr John Reed
Senior Principal Medical Officer
Mental Health Division
Department of Health

Professor Eugene Paykel
Department of Psychiatry
University of Cambridge

Dr Rachel Jenkins
Principal Medical Officer
Mental Health Division
Department of Health

Professor John Wing
Director
Research Unit
The Royal College of Psychiatrists

Dr David Melzer
Senior Registrar in Public Health Medicine
West Lambeth Health Authority

Dr Sheila Adam
Public Health Director
North West Thames Regional Health Authority

Introduction

Dr John Reed

This book is the product of a series of two workshops held in Autumn 1990 sponsored by the Department of Health, and organised by Dr Rachel Jenkins of the Department of Health and the Royal College of Psychiatrists and by Dr Sian Griffiths of the Faculty of Public Health Medicine. They take a look at the issue of how the Annual Reports of the Directors of Public Health can comment on mental health in their populations, on identification of need, and on assessment of outcome of care. We were particularly keen to promote collaboration between Directors of Public Health and psychiatrists, and therefore we invited all the Directors of Public Heatlth, and asked them to identify a suitable psychiatrist to bring with them, and indeed offered a reduced rate for such joint bookings! In the event, we had 29 pairs of joint attendances on day 1 and 33 pairs on day 2.

The first day concentrated on defining needs and Dr Farrow, from the Health Care Evaluation Unit at Bristol University, started the day off by telling us that of 133 district reports analysed by 31st March 1990, only 13 gave any information at all on mental health, and of 7 regional reports, only 2 reported on mental health. Dr Farrow drew the clear conclusion that mental health was neglected as a topic, and that even where mental illness was mentioned, it focused on hospital processes (eg admissions) rather than on prevalence rates in the community. Furthermore there was no evaluation of the outcome of mental health care. Professor Anthony Mann from the Institute of Psychiatry then outlined the epidemiology of the different categories of mental illness, and emphasised the major public health problems of depression and anxiety in adults, dementia in the elderly, and chronic psychotic illness, particularly schizophrenia. Dr Giles Glover gave us a quick resume of the official data available on mental health, which is largely that derived from health service activities (ie processes) eg hospital admissions, and Dr Alastair Macdonald tackled the principles of psychiatric epidemiological measurement. Professor David Goldberg discussed his model of the filters to psychiatric care, which emphasises that it is largely to the community that we must look for empirical data on the mental health needs of the population. Dr Ruaridh Milne described the experiences of Milton Keynes District on behalf of Dr Alison Hill, and Dr Dinshaw Master set out how Guys have started to contract for mental health.

The second day began with Professor Eugene Paykel who bridged that important space between defining needs and measuring outcomes by describing a blueprint for a comprehensive mental health service and some of its key objectives. This was followed by a paper by Dr Rachel Jenkins setting out the key theoretical and practical issues around health care outcome indicators, and proposing a system of indicators of health care input, process and outcome for the major categories of mental illness, including schizophrenia, affective psychosis, neurosis, dementia, mental handicap, child psychiatry, forensic psychiatry, alcohol and drugs. It is hoped that this will form a basis for development by clinicians, researchers and planners for their own requirements. This was followed by Professor John Wing who described plans for audit in mental health by the Royal College of Psychiatrists. Dr David Melzer then gave us details of a local service evaluation in West Lambeth which measured the clinical states, disabilities, social circumstances and use of services by discharged patients with schizophrenia, and described how such data can be used to improve the targeting and co-ordination of services. Dr Sheila Adam concluded the plenary sessions by exploring the implications for Public Health of the NHS Reforms in the light of the new pivotal positions of Directors of Public Health, both in general terms and in relation to mental health. Each day concluded with a number of discussion groups which are reported at the end of each workshop.

One of the overwhelming issues to emerge from the discussions through the day was just how hungry Directors of Public Health are for basic factual epidemiological information about mental health. There was much taking down of references, and pleas for the conferences to be published as soon as possible, which we have now achieved, thanks to HMSO. Public health doctors were heard to mutter 'Why do psychiatrists publish in obscure journals?' Of course, the British Journal of Psychiatry and Psychological Medicine, where most of our work appears, are not obscure to psychiatrists, but we recognise that they are not routine reading for physicians. I think there is a major unsolved difficulty of how public health doctors can keep abreast of key psychiatric research.

Introduction to Annual Reports of the Public Health

Dr Stephen Farrow

Abstract

It is obvious from the broad definition of public health offered by its practitioners at Regional and District level in England that mental health should be as important as physical health.

Nevertheless, of the 133 district annual reports that were analysed, only 13 made any mention of mental health. Of these there was some diversity of content and style. Some reference was made to key indicators used for measuring the prevalence of mental illness. These included the number of admissions to psychiatric hospitals, the number of compulsory admissions under the Mental Health Act, the suicide rate, and alcoholism and drug abuse.

There was some reference in a few reports to the association of socio-economic and cultural factors with mental illness; eg age, sex, marital status, ethnicity, housing conditions, unemployment, immigration, social class and social isolation.

No attempt was made to evaluate the quality and performance of health services in relation to mental health, and only in one district was there an evaluation of process measures, eg bed usage, outpatient attendance and numbers of staff.

Despite the lack of formal evaluation, a number of districts do produce recommendations for mental health. These fall into the broad categories of needs assessment, active prevention, early intervention and appropriateness of care.

In drawing conclusions from the 1989 reports it is important to recognize the possibility that some topics were excluded because they had been extensively covered the previous year. Nevertheless, it does appear that there is extensive undercoverage of mental illness, a general lack of guidelines, a total lack of evaluation, and underdevelopment of mental illness policy.

Introduction

In March 1990 the Department of Health commissioned a review of the District and Regional Annual Public Health Reports. This was carried out over a three month period by the Health Care Evaluation Unit in the Department of Epidemiology and Public Health Medicine in the University of Bristol and an attempt was made to provide an index of the content of the reports so that key words and subjects could be easily accessed. A written review, together with a data base held on floppy discs, has recently been published.[1] The purpose of the review was not to evaluate or rank the reports but to provide an information base on the scope and content of reports across the country as a whole which could be fed back to Directors of Public Health, for use by them in preparing future reports. It was decided by a Steering Group that the review should be attempted, in the first instance, from the most recent report issued by districts and regions by 31 March 1990. This meant that a number of features, for example, the objectives of the report, the intended audience, the size of the print run and the impact of the report would almost certainly not be known to the reviewer. Of the 133 district reports analysed, 22 were dated 1988, 98 were dated 1989 and 13 were dated 1990. Several regional reports, all dated 1990, were available for analysis.

The review was conducted without contact with individual districts and so it was not possible to describe the objectives, the intended audience nor to assess the reports' impact. In reviewing the most recent report available it was not always clear whether this was the district's first, second or third report, nor was it clear whether the narrow focus of some reports was intentional. Data abstraction was carried out by several researchers and despite attempts to reduce inter-observer and intra-observer bias, this will inevitably have occurred. It would be wise to treat the absence of an item within the data set with caution as it may have been missed by the researchers. The genuine omission of a particular item cannot be taken to imply criticism. Without a clear statement of the objectives of a particular report, and without knowing the place of a report in a possible series, any inferences about the significance of a particular omission must be drawn with care. Moreover, certain guide-lines from the Department of Health and from the Faculty of Public Health Medicine may have arrived after district reports were published.[2,4] Issues such as audit, evaluation and the specification of contracts were gaining in perceived importance during 1989 and 1990 and may not have been critical at the time that reports were being written. The range of resources available in individual districts was varied, with a number of districts severely handicapped by inadequate numbers of public health medicine and other staff.

The reports displayed considerable variation and range of content, style and presentation. A number of districts either structured their reports or gave prominence to the following themes: WHO targets; inequalities; working together (with local authorities and voluntary bodies); involving the community. A few districts undertook their own lifestyle or other community surveys. The standard of presentation of many reports was high with extensive use of graphics, charts, histograms, photographs and maps. However, there was a relative lack of attention given to the physically handicapped; the mentally ill; the mentally handicapped; and to primary care. There was little evidence of the application of modern techniques to the study of the assessment of needs and to the evaluation of the effectiveness and the quality of care. The standards of publication were generally low with no district report having an index and several failing to have a simple table of contents. Few districts produced their reports in different formats for different audiences. In general the annual reports appeared not to have exploited fully the potential for advocating change and influencing the delivery of health care and the promotion of health.

Coverage of mental health in District Annual Reports

Despite the limitations of the review process an attempt has been made to use the data base to review the way in which directors of public health have addressed the issue of mental health. It is obvious that the definition of public health used in most reports does imply that mental health should be as important to the individual as physical health. Nevertheless the coverage of mental health was relatively poor. Of the 133 districts being analysed, only 13 gave information about mental health. They were Barking Havering & Brentwood, Bristol & Weston, Ealing, East Surrey, North Bedfordshire, Plymouth, Redbridge, Riverside, Southend, Walsall, Waltham Forest, West Birmingham and West Surrey. Of the 7 regions analysed only 2 reported on mental health, South East Thames and Trent. In the following section an attempt will be made to draw attention to some of the features emerging in these reports concerning mental illness. It will cover the key indicators used for measuring mental illness; associated socio-economic and cultural factors; the evaluation of quality and performance; and recommendations made by districts.

Admissions to psychiatric hospitals were used by most of the health authorities. Some used this indicator as a proxy for the prevalence of mental disorder, although in most cases it was suggested that this would result in an underestimate because many patients were treated by their GPs and are only rarely admitted to hospitals. It was also indicated by several health districts that the number of admissions was a measure of events not of people. A second indicator, the number of compulsory admissions under the Mental Health Act, was reported by three districts. Suicide rates were used by several districts although this was usually accompanied by a caveat that the relationship between suicide rates and population rates of mental illness was not clearly established. It was argued by some districts that alcoholism and drug abuse gave some indication of the prevalence of mental illness. Although all four indicators were of some value none gave a good measure of the incidence and prevalence of mental disorder in patients presenting to their GPs.

Some districts reported a relationship between the prevalence of mental illness and factors such as age, sex, marital status, ethnicity, housing condition, unemployment, migration, social class and social isolation. Barking, Havering and Brentwood reported a relatively high hospitalisation rate for elderly people with mental illness which was above the national average. Walsall and Ealing drew attention to higher rates of attendance amongst women. In Ealing female attenders outnumbered males at every age in its three Mental Health Resource Centres. It was argued that this might be a function of the acceptability and availability of these services to women. The question of marital status was considered by Walsall who noted that single men were more at risk than married and the reverse was true for women. Riverside and West Birmingham commented on the disproportionately high schizophrenia rate amongst some ethnic groups. West Birmingham also commented that Asians were under-represented as users of the mental health service. A further conclusion from West Birmingham concerned housing conditions where the high density of people in multi-occupied properties was associated with high treatment rates for serious mental illness. The Bristol and Weston District reported a great difference in admission rates from the deprived city areas of Bristol compared to rural areas and drew attention to the association with various indicators of deprivation including the high rate of unemployment. Other factors, including migration, social class and social isolation, were mentioned by one or two districts but no detailed statistics were presented.

Most of the districts offered information on the services provided locally, from health authorities, local authorities and voluntary bodies. However, they failed to address the limitations of the mental health service and did not discuss the unmet needs of customers. Only Ealing attempted to evaluate the performance of health services by using indicators of bed usage in inpatient services, average attendances in outpatient services and information on staffing levels. Figures were given that showed where Ealing lay in relation to the national averages for those indicators. No district evaluated the outcome, quality or cost-effectiveness of the mental illness services.

Approximately half of those districts that had made reference to mental health in their annual report also made recommendations about their aims and future plans. In general the recommendations fell into four areas.

(i) **The assessment of needs.** It was recommended that more information should be collected on the use of services so that they could be made more appropriate and acceptable. The establishment of case registers would provide valuable information for health service managers and would ensure that patients were not lost to the service. More attention should be given to the needs of carers, both formal and informal.

(ii) **Active prevention.** Individual and social coping mechanisms should be reinforced to reduce the negative consequence of threat and loss (such as bereavement or unemployment). The availability of help at an early stage could prevent problems from developing or worsening.

(iii) **Early intervention.** Services to reduce the incidence and level of alcohol or drug dependence should be developed, including detoxification. Services for those attempting suicide and other forms of self harm should be encouraged. Maintenance and treatment should be provided at home, thus reducing the need for hospital admissions and re-admissions.

(iv) **Appropriateness of care.** Various ways of enabling consumers to express their views about the services they receive should be developed. Greater emphasis would be given to the resettlement of patients from hospitals into the community with the help of Local Authorities and voluntary bodies. Joint financing and joint care planning should be further developed. Facilities for the elderly mentally ill should be provided separately to meet the particular needs of this group in a more home-like setting. Nurse staffing levels in hospitals should be increased.

Coverage of mental health in Regional Annual Reports

Of the seven regions analysed, only 2 reported the mental health of their own regional population. They were South East Thames and Trent and both addressed the issue in great detail.

The South East Thames report provided an outstanding discussion of the mental health services in its region. It had several unique features, including an overview of the incidence and prevalence of psychiatric disorder which other reports had not achieved. It reported not only the number of first admissions to psychiatric hospital, but also information about the prevalence of untreated mental illness obtained from the Camberwell Community Survey. It was the only report which described extensively the evaluative studies concerning the quality of life of those discharged from hospital to community-based care and the impact of the hospital closure programme on the wider development of community care. For example, the closure of Cane Hill Hospital was investigated by two groups of researchers who looked into the general life of patients both before and after discharge; the suitability of some forms of placement in the community; the need for 24 hour care; and the shift of resource allocation and its implications. It gave a brief evaluation of the cost effectiveness of its policy, including the costs of staff recruitment and retraining and the financial consequences of the acquisition of land, the conversion of new premises and the disposal of redundant hospital sites.

The Trent report was titled 'Hearts and Minds' and looked in detail at coronary heart disease and mental disorders. With regard to mental illness the following areas were covered: the prevalence of different types of mental health problems including schizophrenia, affective psychoses, neuroses, suicide and senile dementia; the inadequacy of statistics about the use of services which did not include people who were in non-psychiatric hospitals and did not take account of the resources used in the community; the cost of mental health problems for the patient, the family, the community and the health service. The recommendations made in this report were generally similar in approach to those in the district reports.

Conclusions

Despite the limitations of the review process and the possibility that districts had either tackled the subject of mental health in a previous report or were planning coverage in some future report it is possible to draw some general conclusions. They fall broadly into four areas.

Undercoverage of mental illness

On the whole, mental health appeared to be neglected as a topic. In those reports that did discuss mental illness, there was an under-reporting of its prevalence in the community.

Lack of guidelines

In general, there was a lack of guidelines on how to compile and assemble mental health data. This problem has not yet been adequately addressed. The Acheson Report[5] and the latest edition of the Health Measurement Toolbox[6] did not provide guide-lines on how to report mental health services.

Lack of evaulation

Health Authorities have not yet managed to evaluate the outcome of mental health care. Some evidence of process evaluation is available but this is rare.

Lack of policy

Few Health Authorities attempted to provide strategic plans for the development of mental health services.

References

[1] Farrow S C, Wood N, Beattie A. A content review of the annual reports on the health of the population. Bristol: Health Care Evaluation Unit, University of Bristol; 1990.

[2] Department of Health. Annual reports on the health of the population. Circular EL(89)P/203. London: Department of Health; 1989.

[3] Faculty of Community Medicine. Report of the working party on annual reports of directors of public health. London: Faculty of Community Medicine; 1989.

[4] Faculty of Community Medicine. Health measurement toolbox: measuring health for the annual report. London: Faculty of Community Medicine; 1989.

[5] Report of the Committee of Enquiry into the future development of the Public Health Function (Acheson Report). Public Health in England. London: HMSO; 1988.

[6] Faculty of Public Health Medicine. Health measurement toolbox: measuring health for the annual report. London: Faculty of Public Health Medicine; 1990.

Public Health and Psychiatric Morbidity

Professor Anthony Mann

Abstract

The public health doctor will be concerned with mental illness as it affects the whole population in the district as well as with the effective delivery of care to those sufferers who have made contact with service providers. The latter providers are the formal psychiatric services (approximately 8,000 contacts per year/100,000) and the general practitioners (approximately 22,000 contacts per year/100,000).

The work of the formal psychiatric services has been effectively monitored by the use of case registers over the last 20 years. Data from one such (Salford) will be presented that suggests that schizophrenia represents a constant burden, but also shows that contacts for depression and dementia are increasing. The biggest increase in new contacts with the psychiatric services over the last decade has come from those over 75.

The family doctor predominantly sees patients with neurotic disorders and can expect to manage 300 such per year. Many of these conditions become chronic. It has also been shown from research studies that approximately one third of consultations may have a significant psychiatric component to the clinical picture, but this may not always be recognised.

Community surveys suggest the prevalence of schizophrenia is under 1%, and that the majority of community cases are known to the psychiatric services or the general practitioner. More common, as discovered by community surveys, are the syndromes of depression and anxiety (9% approximately at case level), but also it seems that symptoms of depression, anxiety and fatigue, etc. are very prevalent, reported by up to a third of the population. There are no adequate data at the moment on the precise diagnoses, the burden and personal distress, nor the service use, from individuals with these complaints.

Community surveys also suggest that alcohol intake, particularly in men, is above 'safe' levels for those who report themselves as moderate drinkers. Again, precise data on the implications for this in terms of personal damage, service use and economic cost, is missing.

There is a high level of psychiatric morbidity amongst the over 65s. 6% approximately suffer from dementia and 15% from clinical depression. Many fewer of these sufferers are known to formal psychiatric services or to general practitioners than is the case with the younger adult with mental illness.

Consultations

A doctor in public health might begin to understand the distribution of mental illness in his or her district by seeing where the activity lies, ie, where mental health consultations are taking place.

Table 1 shows consultations for mental disorders classifiable under the Mental Disorder Section of ICD9. These rates are shown per 100,000 of the population. (Where possible all figures presented in this paper will refer to a district containing 100,000 people). It can be seen that 2½ times the number of consultations take place in the surgeries of the 40 or so general practitioners in the district than do in the totality of the psychiatric services.

Table 1 Comparative rates of attendance for different levels of psychiatric care (rates per 100,000 general population, all ages and sexes combined in 1981)

	General practitioner consultations*	Out-patients attendances†	Day hospital attendances†	Psychiatric admissions†
ICD–9 290–315 Mental Disorders	22,980	3,532	4,943	397

*Obtained from: Morbidity Statistics from General Practice 1981–1982.
†Obtained from: Mental Health Enquiry for England, 1981

(Sharp D, Morrell D (1989) The Psychiatry of General Practice. In: Scope of Epidemiological Psychiatry. Routledge).

This disparity, however, might be a great surprise, but ought not to be, for many more people with other chronic conditions–arthritis, hypertension or diabetes–must be being managed by their general practitioners than hospital doctors. From these statistics, the doctor might proceed (i) to look for more specific data of the type of conditions being seen within the psychiatric services and by general practitioners. (ii) to discover what is known about mental illness in the community itself and the relationship of these identified consultations, that represent the therapeutic work of the professional groups in the district, to the needs of the mentally ill in the community.

The Psychiatric Services

A most valuable resource in monitoring the case load of the psychiatric services, and changes therein over the years, has been the case register. These are local information systems that record contacts with designated medical and social services by patients from a defined geographic area. As the data is recorded by professionals, it is likely to be of high quality. Such registers, however, do not of course detect what is going on in the general practitioner's surgery, nor provide information on those mentally ill not making contact. Further, they cannot determine whether a cessation of a contact means that the patient has left the district or is just remaining unwell at home and out of reach of the services. An example of an inner city register, is that in Salford. This register was set up by Fryers and colleagues, in 1974, in an area serving about ¼ million people near Manchester. The register began in the inner city area of Salford East and then added on the more suburban Salford West later. The contact data consist of those made by patients with psychiatrists, nurses and mental health social workers from the defined Salford area.

Table 2 shows point prevalence rates of cases of various psychiatric disorders known on 1st January on each of several years of the register's life. Included are patients who are inpatients or day patients on the census day and outpatient contacts, if they had occurred within three months around census date. The Table shows that Salford has about 700 schizophrenic patients in contact out of 100,000 of the population. This number seems to have been constant over the years. Over this time, there has been a rise in frequency of contact by other patients with diagnoses: depression, dementia, anxiety, personality disorder and alcoholism. The rise in these diagnoses seems to have been greater among females than males. Particularly striking are the numbers of female patients with dementia, rising from 56/100,000 to 186/100,000, over this 10 year period.

Table 3 shows the prevalence trends according to age bands. There has been a noticeable jump in contacts by those over 75 over these 10 years. It

Table 2 Salford: Point prevalence on 1 January for all services, 1976–87. Numbers and rates per 1,000 adult population: sex and diagnosis

Diagnosis	1976		1979		1983		1987	
	No.	Rate	No.	Rate	No.	Rate	No.	Rate
Schizophrenias								
Male	311	3.22	345	3.66	347	3.64	343	3.70
Female	340	2.87	345	3.34	358	3.49	332	3.32
Depressions								
Male	98	1.02	165	1.75	195	2.05	201	2.17
Female	252	2.38	375	3.63	514	5.01	594	5.95
Dementias								
Male	20	0.21	49	0.52	48	0.50	60	0.65
Female	59	0.56	113	1.09	137	1.34	186	1.86
Others								
Male	156	1.62	225	2.39	330	3.47	409	4.42
Female	192	1.81	277	2.68	456	4.44	543	5.44
Total								
Male	**585**	**6.06**	**784**	**8.32**	**920**	**9.66**	**1,013**	**10.94**
Female	**807**	**7.63**	**1,110**	**10.75**	**1,465**	**14.28**	**1,655**	**16.53**

From: Health Service Planning & Research. Ed. J K Wing, Gaskell (1989)

Table 3 Year prevalence (all Salford services) 1976–86. Age-specific rates per 1,000 population

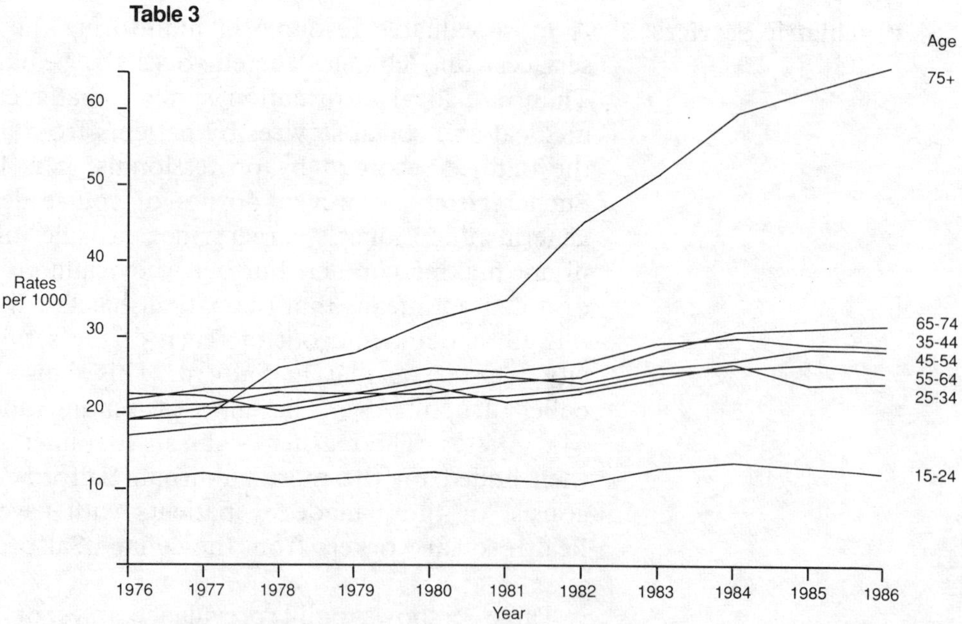

Year prevalence (all Salford services) 1976-86. Age-specific rates per 1000 population

From: Health Service Planning & Research. Ed. J K Wing, Gaskell (1989)

appears that in 1981, a new specialist psychogeriatrician was appointed, but the trend of increased contact for this age group seems to have started before that date. Inception rates from the Salford register–contacts by patients with no previous contact–shows a similar steady rate for each diagnosis. The exception were new contacts with the register by the very old, these quadrupling over the 10 year period.

There have been other excellent registers–Camberwell, Southampton, Nottingham and Worcester. However, central support for these registers has now been withdrawn as each district is required to collect its own service data.

The Primary Care Sector

What sort of problems are provided by mental illness for the general practitioner? Table 4 indicates the scale of mental illness work undertaken by general practitioners, as can be determined from the National Morbidity Statistics, based upon returns of collaborating practices on the frequency and reason for these consultations. One limitation of these statistics is that the diagnoses are made by the general practitioners (possibly a problem in this area); psychiatric disorder may be not recognised by a general practitioner and so not recorded. However, with the aid of research studies conducted by teams under Professors Michael Shepherd and David Goldberg over the last 20 years, information about primary care psychiatry is fairly sophisticated.

Table 4 Psychiatric Morbidity in Primary Care

(1)	1980	Consultations (National Morbidity Statistics)		
	Reason:	Respiratory System	15.4%	
		Circulatory System	11.2%	
		Mental Disorders	9.6%	
(2)	Prevalence rate	140/1,000 at risk		
	Inception rate	52/1,000		[Shepherd *et al* 1966]
		GP may manage 300 cases/year		
(3)	Tendency to Chronicity			
	Approximately 50% lasting for one year			[Mann *et al* 1981]

Psychiatric disorders represent the third commonest reason for consultations. The typical consulters with psychiatric disorders are the middle-aged, between 25–55, and women consult for recognised disorders 2½ more times as men. Surprisingly, the old, as judged by the morbidity statistics, seem rather infrequent consulters for psychiatric disorders, but this finding might reflect a particular recognition problem of psychiatric morbidity in this age group. Shepherd's original study in 1966 of the psychiatric morbidity in general practice, suggested that the 'average' general practitioner may recognise and manage 300 cases per year. Psychiatry-related consultations however are even more frequent, perhaps up to a third of all consultations in primary care, although many are not so recognised. As with the illnesses seen by psychiatrists, the psychiatric disorders in preliminary care can become chronic, for follow-up studies indicate that 50% of patients who consult their general practitioner with a psychiatric disorder are still symptomatic at one year, 20–25% still symptomatic at three years.

Table 5 provides details of the type and relative frequency of each type of psychiatric disorder as seen by the general practitioner. There is a relative rarity of the psychoses–the major psychiatric syndromes of schizophrenia and dementia–and an overwhelming preponderance of the neurotic disorders.

There is thus evidence of two styles of psychiatric activity going on in a district. What is the relationship of either to the actual morbidity in the community itself?

Community Survey Data

There are two approaches to detecting morbidity in the population. The first draws a sampling frame that represents the whole and screens this sample with an instrument that allows all forms of psychiatric morbidity to be detected. The second concentrates specifically on one disorder thereby

Table 5 Psychiatric disorder and social pathology in an average general practice population of 2,500

Acute major disorders	Cases per annum
Severe depression	12
Suicide attempts	3
Completed suicide	One every three years
Chronic mental illness	55
Severe mental handicap	10
Neurotic disorders	300
Social pathology	
Chronic alcoholism (known cases)	5
Chronic alcoholism (unknown cases)	25
Juvenile delinquency	5–7
Problem families	5–10
Broken homes (one-parent families with children under 15)	60

From: Royal College of General Practitioners (1973).

Table 6 Camden Schizophrenia Survey

South Camden (530 individuals)

- Point Prevalence 0.98%
  980 Cases/1,000,000
- 20% inpatient } 69%
- 49% psychiatric services }
- 15% homeless hostels
- 25% GP alone

North Camden (590 individuals)

- Point Prevalence 0.56%
- 560 Cases/100,000

- 14% inpatient } 66%
- 52% psychiatric services }
- 23% GP alone

From: Campbell P G *et al* (1990). International Perspectives in Schizophrenia. Ed. Weller M (Libbey).

adopting a case-finding strategy that most effectively seeks out that condition. The Camden Schizophrenia Survey (Table 6) is an example of the second approach. On two separate census days in 1985 and 1986 in South and North Camden respectively, all individuals of 18 or over with a probable diagnosis of schizophrenia were identified from any health or social service agency in the district including primary care settings. Some patients, for example vagrants, will have been missed, but it is efficient for a relatively rare condition that tends to cause disturbance and hence is unlikely to be left undetected.

The results of this enumeration were as follows: the point prevalence rates were 0.56 and 0.98–higher in South Camden, perhaps because of its closeness to a major rail terminal. What is striking is that between a fifth and a sixth of the samples were currently inpatients or day patients, about half of them were living in the community and in current contact with some arm of the psychiatric service, and a quarter being managed by the general practitioner alone. As the authors felt they had a reasonably complete view of schizophrenia, they related prevalence rates to the Jarman indices of social deprivation by electoral ward. The result was a strong significant relationship between the prevalence rate of schizophrenia and higher indices of social deprivation.

This method of community research can be contrasted with that used by Bebbington and colleagues in Camberwell (Table 7). A sample of 800 individuals were chosen from the electoral roll, screened and then followed up for assessment using the Present State Examination. Diagnoses were thus obtained and the number of individuals reaching PSE criteria for 'caseness' became the basis of the prevalence figures. The general survey showed that psychotic patients were rare compared to other disorders.

Table 7 Prevalence of Psychiatric Disorders. Age 18–64 in 1980 in Camberwell (derived from PSE)

ICD 9	Male %	Female %	Total %
Psychosis	0.3		**0.2**
Manic Depressive: Mania		1.4	**0.8**
Depression: Reactive & Endogenous	4.8	9.0	**7.0**
Anxiety, Phobia, Obsessional Disorders	1.0	4.5	**2.9**

From: Bebbington *et al* 1981. Psychological Medicine, 11, p. 561–579

This very low prevalence for psychosis confirms that if the interest of a survey is the distribution and associated factors of schizophrenia or other psychoses in the community, then the method adopted in the Camden survey is a more realistic one.

The majority of cases detected by the PSE were in the diagnostic categories of depression or anxiety. However, the concept of 'caseness' used by this instrument was artificial, for the criteria of caseness here is a cut off on a continuum of complaint. The level at which this cut-off occurs is that at which psychiatrists would agree that symptoms are sufficiently persistent and intrusive for intervention to be necessary. However, the prevalence of the actual symptom or complaint of depression or anxiety is much greater than this, as indicated by results from a recent total survey of the United Kingdom population, The Health and Lifestyle Survey. A random sample of 9,000 individuals were interviewed throughout the United Kingdom.

Table 8 Scores on 30-item General Health Questionnaire by age and sex.

	Age 18–24	25–34	35–44	45–54	55–64	65–74	75+	All ages
Percentage scoring 5+ (ie above the recommended threshold value, 4/5)								
Males	30	28	24	27	26	25	39	27
Females	38	34	28	35	31	33	43	33
Both sexes	34	31	26	32	29	29	41	31
Base = 100%								
Males	*365*	*538*	*566*	*442*	*489*	*336*	*148*	*2,892*
Females	*426*	*741*	*777*	*585*	*534*	*380*	*171*	*3,606*
Both sexes	*791*	*1,279*	*1,343*	*1,027*	*1,023*	*716*	*319*	*6,498*

From: Huppert F A *et al.* In: Health & Lifestyle Survey, Preliminary Report, Health Promotion Research Trust [1987]

Table 8 shows that, from that survey, approximately a quarter of men and a third of women gave a positive response to the General Health Questionnaire, a screening instrument that identifies probable cases of psychiatric morbidity. The frequency of specific 'psychiatric' complaints were also detected in the same survey, eg insomnia, fatigue, nerves, these being reported between a fifth and a quarter of the population.

Table 9 Incidence of specific symptoms of Malaise 'during the last month' by age

Malaise symptom	Age 18–24	25–34	35–44	45–54	55–64	65–74	75+
	Percentage						
Males							
Difficulty sleeping	19	20	18	20	22	22	26
Always feeling tired	22	19	19	17	19	15	23
Worrying over every little thing	14	12	12	14	16	10	15
Nerves	6	5	5	7	8	6	7
Difficulty concentrating	13	10	9	10	10	10	14
Often or always bored	3	5	9	8	7	4	2
Often or always lonely	16	11	8	9	12	9	13
Often or always 'under so much strain that your health is likely to suffer'	3	3	2	4	5	8	14
Base = 100%	*535*	*724*	*745*	*594*	*628*	*448*	*231*
Females							
Difficulty sleeping	23	24	21	38	39	42	40
Always feeling tired	34	33	32	29	25	25	28
Worrying over every little thing	26	24	23	33	30	30	25
Nerves	12	9	12	17	16	17	15
Difficulty concentrating	14	11	14	18	17	17	17
Often or always bored	5	6	8	9	6	6	6
Often or always lonely	19	14	7	10	9	12	15
Often or always 'under so much strain that your health is likely to suffer'	9	7	7	8	8	12	17
Base = 100%	*625*	*976*	*1,007*	*792*	*762*	*592*	*344*

From: Stark J. In: Health & Lifestyle Survey, Preliminary Report, Health Promotion Research Trust [1987]

Thus while caseness, as suggested by the PSE, is around 10%, complaints of symptoms that constitute the diagnostic syndrome of anxiety or depressive neurosis, seem to be very much commoner. Unfortunately there is a major gap so far as public health knowledge is concerned, in that there is no information on the degree of handicap, service use, or economic wastage for individuals with such complaints. The consultations for neurosis in primary care and the large volume of prescriptions for tranquillisers and antidepressants by general practitioners, are clearly one effect. There is a great deal of 'low grade' psychiatric morbidity, which we cannot define very accurately (Table 9).

The Health and Lifestyle Survey also shows some other rather disturbing data not unrelated to the previous complaints. This was the reported alcohol consumption of their sample in a UK population. Respondents to this survey were asked to rate themselves according to their own classification of their drinking habit and to keep a diary of their alcohol intake over the last week. Such data are imperfect, but nevertheless provided some worrying statistics. Light or moderate drinking seems to be the norm for men, while this is less so for women and for the older people in the survey (Table 10).

However, Table 11 shows what respondents mean by these self-rated categories in terms of the number of units they have recorded consuming in the past week. The mean number of units reported by moderate drinking men is well over the 'safe' limits of 21 units per week. Women moderate drinkers seem 'safer', their mean consumption being lower than the 14 units recommended for them. These safe limits are, of course, very general criteria and not an absolute guarantee of freedom from harm from alcohol.

Table 10 Categories of drinker by age and sex

	Males			Females		
	Age 18–39	40–59	60+	18–39	40–59	60+
	Percentage					
Always non-drinker or only very occasional	8	13	22	23	32	54
Ex-drinker	5	8	10	6	5	5
Regular drinker:						
none 'last week'	9	11	9	17	11	9
light	27	23	35	27	28	19
moderate	44	40	22	27	24	14
heavy	8	5	3	1	0	0
Base = 100%	*1,668*	*1,240*	*997*	*2,150*	*1,596*	*1,352*

From: Blaxter M. In: The Health & Lifestyle Survey, Preliminary Report, Health Promotion Research Trust [1987]

Table 11 Own definition of drinking and actual amount (mean units in last week)

	Male			Female		
	Light	Moderate	Heavy	Light	Moderate	Heavy
Age	(1,465)	(1,506)	(144)	(1,973)	(1,085)	(24)
18/39	10.03	27.46	52.88	4.92	10.95	21.55
40/59	9.42	25.73	53.41	4.68	10.28	16.57
60+	7.77	23.15	39.42	4.88	10.27	

From: Blaxter M. In: The Health and Lifestyle Survey, Preliminary Report, Health Promotion Research Trust [1987]

There is another unfortunate gap here, for there is no recent community survey in the United Kingdom on the effects of this large alcohol intake, ie the drinking pattern, the mental, physical, and social sequelae, and the service use of these people. For instance, how many of these 'moderate' male drinkers are consulting in medical outpatients with non-specific gastro-intestinal complaints?

The Older Population

What of the future? Population trends indicate the ageing of the United Kingdom's as well as other Western European populations. At the moment, 21% of the United Kingdom population is over 60, a proportion rising to about 26% in 50 years time. However, within this age band there is a change in the relative proportion of the old old to the young old. In 1985, there were some 700,000 people over 85 representing 6% of the over 60's. These will increase by 50% to reach 1,100,000 by the end of the century (Table 12). An ageing population brings with it many pressing problems. Very old age brings with it high rates of physical disease, dependency and depression and a rate of dementia that rises to 25% at that age, compared to a prevalence rate of 1% in the 60–65 year old band. The effect of the age change may be already visible in the Salford register data.

To illustrate the current frequency of mental illness in old age, data from a population sample identified by household enumeration of the over 65's, is presented. In one electoral ward in North London in 1987, all pensioners (803) were identified by door-to-door contact. They were then screened to

Table 12 Projections of the elderly population of Great Britain 1985–2041

Age Group	1985		1991		1996		2001		2011		2021		2041	
	m	fm	m	fm	m	fm	m	fm	m	fm	m	fm	m	fm
Standard projection assumptions													hundred-thousands	
60–64	15	17	14	15	13	14	14	14	18	19	18	19	15	15
65–74	22	28	23	28	23	27	22	26	24	27	28	32	29	32
75–84	10	19	12	20	12	20	13	20	13	19	15	20	19	27
85+	2	5	2	7	3	8	3	8	4	9	4	9	6	11
60+	49	69	51	70	51	69	52	68	59	74	65	80	69	85
all ages	276	290	281	294	286	297	290	300	293	301	296	303	292	299

[OPCS (1987) HMSO London]
From: Warnes A M (1989) Elderly people in Great Britain: variable projections and characteristics. Care of the Elderly, Vol. 1, No. 1, 7–10.

detect psychiatric morbidity using a standard interview containing indicator scales. Those whose score suggested depression or dementia were subject to a more detailed Phase 2 assessment.

Table 13 shows the prevalence rates of dementia. The screening scale indicated that memory impairment, without diagnostic import, occurred in about 8%. A more precise scale from that screening instrument classified 4.8% with probable clinical dementia. These respondents tended to be older and female compared to the rest of the population. A subsequent clinical evaluation suggested that the correct rate for all forms of clinical dementia was 6.7%. If this percentage were extrapolated to a population of a 100,000, with 18% elderly, then there would be 1000–1200 people suffering from dementia. This number exceeds the 590 discovered to have schizophrenia in the same district. Probably 10% of these individuals with dementia were known to the psychiatrist and about 25% to the general practitioner, these figures contrasting unfavourably with those shown for schizophrenia.

Table 13 Gospel Oak Study

Prevalence of Dementia (65+)

	Criterion	*Rate*
Phase I —	SHORT CARE	
	Organic Brain Syndrome	8%
	Pervasive Dementia	4.8%
Phase II —	CLINICAL ASSESSMENT	
	All dementia syndromes	6.7%*
	McKhann Probable SDAT	3.0%
	Mixed/MID	0.8%
	Secondary	0.8%
	Unclassified	2.0%

*Estimated numbers of cases in a population of 100,000 (18% over 65) = 1,000–1,200

-Known to GP: possibly 25%
-Known to Psychiatric Services: 5%–10%

Refs. (1) Livingston *et al*, 1990, Psychol. Med., 20, No. 1, 137–146.
(2) Livingston *et al*, 1990, Psychol. Med. (in press).

Table 14 Gospel Oak Study

Prevalence of Depression (65+)

I **SHORT CARE**
Depressive symptoms – 26%
Pervasive depression – 16.1%

II **CLINICAL ASSESSMENT**
(underway)
3/4 cases by Geriatric Mental State*

*Estimated cases in population of 100,000 with 18% elderly = 2,000–3,000

Proportion known to General Practitioner: 10–15%
Proportion known to Psychiatric Services: <5%

A similar picture is shown for depression in the same population (Table 14). A quarter of the population at screening were found to have significantly depressive symptoms, 16% being classified as having depression to a level that intervention should be considered. The latter group are now being assessed in more detail as part of an intervention study. At least ¾ have been shown to definite 'cases' using standard valid diagnostic criteria. Such figures would suggest that there are between 2000–3000 elderly in a population of 100,000 with depression at a level that intervention would be considered necessary. Only a fraction of the depressed old people were known to the general practitioner and to the psychiatric services. These cases of depression and dementia meet diagnostic criteria: not included are forgetfulness or unhappiness, even more common in old age.

Cost

Public health doctors must be aware of the financial implications of mental disorders. As it happens, two reports have emerged recently that have attempted to cost specific conditions. The direct cost of schizophrenia and neurosis seems similar, although the drug costs are higher for the latter condition. Indirect costs in terms of retirement and loss of earnings and, in the case of schizophrenia, premature mortality, are higher for both. However, the sums are estimated as being four times as high for neurosis as for schizophrenia, again reflecting the large numbers of neurotic patients.

Table 15 Costs

Schizophrenia [Davies & Drummond, Brit. J. Psychiatry, 1990]		
• Minimal Cost to Health & Social Services (Drug Costs 3% = £9 million)		= £310 million
• Indirect Costs: Premature Mortality, Early Retirement, Unemployment		= £1,606 million
Neurosis in Primary Care [Croft-Jeffreys & Wilkinson, Psychol. Med. 1989]		
• Minimal Costs		= £373 million
Consultations and Drug Costs	£119.5 million	
Costs of Certified Sickness Absence	£253 million	
• Indirect Costs: Early Retirement		= £2,700 million
Uncertified Sickness Absence		= £2,900 million
		= £5,600 million

Conclusions

1. Mental illness is distributed widely in the population, the formal services and general practitioners are each dealing with a subset containing different disorders. The scale of psychiatric morbidity and of alcohol consumption would indicate that such disorders must be included in public health considerations.
2. The formal psychiatric services are currently in an upheaval with the new policies for community care and relocating patients who would formerly have been in hospital. However, it is important to note that those in hospital represent only a fifth of those with major mental illnesses in the community. Community resources must be devoted to all, rather than those just being devolved from hospital. Schizophrenics, particularly, live in the poorest areas in a community, thereby indicating where community resources should be sited, but also implying that they are exposed to many social disadvantages. However, register data suggests that prevalence rates of these major mental illnesses seem to be stable and research data suggests the majority of these patients are known to the services. The resource demand for this component of the mental health services should perhaps become finite.
3. In contrast, the older aged in the population are growing in number and show high and apparently undetected rates of mental illness. If psychiatric services are to expand, then perhaps they ought preferentially to do so in the areas of old age psychiatry. With the creation of the speciality of old age psychiatry there have been important developments over the last 10 years.
4. There seems to be no detailed data on the very common 'neurotic' disorders which are widespread in the population, and on the impact they have on personal happiness, economic activity and on the use of services. There is a similar lack of data on the consequences of the apparently large volume of alcohol being consumed. Both these, because of their frequency, must be potential drains on the health of the community. While primary care obviously deals with many such patients, it is not known what proportion of the problem is tackled and how effective that intervention is. There is a need for more information in this area. At the current time, it is not clear who is going to take up this challenge. Will it be the psychiatrist, who is more than ever preoccupied with the major mental illnesses, or the general practitioner who now has new pressures on his time and a relative lack of training in mental illness research, or should it be the public health doctor?

References

Bebbington P, Hurry J, Tennant C, Sturt E & Wing J K (1981). Epidemiology of mental disorders in Camberwell. Psychological Medicine, 11: 561–579.

Blaxter M (1987). Alcohol Consumption. In: Health & Lifestyle Survey, Prelimary Report. Promotion Research Trust, 109–119.

Campbell P G, Taylor J, Pantelis C & Harvey C (1990). Studies of schizophrenia in a large mental hospital proposed for closure, and in two halves of an inner London borough served by the hospital. In: International Perspectives in Schizophrenia. (Ed M Weller). London: John Libbey, 185–202.

Croft-Jeffreys C & Wilkinson G (1989). Estimated costs of neurotic disorder in UK general practice 1985. Psychological Medicine, 19, 549–558.

Davies L M & Drummond M F (1990). The economic burden of schizophrenia. Bulletin of the British Journal of Psychiatry, 14, 522–525.

Fryers T & Wooff K (1989). A decade of mental health care in an English urban community: patterns and trends in Salford, 1976–87, In: Health Service Planning & Research (Ed J K Wing). London: Gaskell, 31–52.

Huppert F A, Roth M & Gore M (1987). Psychological Factors. In: Health & Lifestyle Survey, Preliminary Report. Promotion Research Trust, 51–58.

Livingston G, Hawkins A, Graham N, Blizard R & Mann A H (1990). The Gospel Oak Study: Prevalence rates of dementia, depression and activity limitation among elderly residents in inner London. Psychological Medicine, 20, No 1, 137–146.

Livingston G, Sax K, Willison J, Blizard R & Mann A H (1990). The Gospel Oak Project Stage 2: The diagnosis of dementia in the community. Psychological Medicine, 20: 881–892.

Mann A H, Jenkins R & Belsey E (1981). The twelve-month outcome of patients with neurotic illness in general practice. Psychological Medicine, 11: 535–550.

Royal College of General Practitioners (1973). National Morbidity Statistics. London: HMSO.

Shepherd M, Cooper B, Brown A C & Kalton G (1966). Psychiatric Illness in General Practice. Oxford: Oxford University Press

Sharp D & Morrell D (1989). The Psychiatry of General Practice. In: Scope for Epidemiological Psychiatry (Eds P Williams, G Wilkinson & K Rawnsley). London: Routledge pp. 404–419

Stark J. (1987). Health and Social Contacts. In: Health & Lifestyle Survey, Preliminary Report. Health Promotion Research Trust, 59–66.

Warnes A M (1989). Elderly people in Great Britain: variable projections and characteristics. Care of the Elderly, Vol 1, No 1, 7–10

The Official Data Available on Mental Health

Dr Gyles Glover

Abstract

Needs for mental health services are currently of interest both in the process of specifying service contracts and in compiling public health reports. There are problems in attempting to assess these needs from official data sources which give district specific data for all of England and Wales. Data about health service usage provides only a partial view of NHS services. The data is at present seriously incomplete and there are concerns about its reliability.

In different districts the health authority, local authority and voluntary sectors undertake different components of the work. Thus a picture from available official statistics does not provide straightforward cross-district comparisons. Nonetheless, suitably critical analysis of several data sets can give an insight into features of local services. Examples given include detailed analysis of stay-length distributions, occupancy rates, and service use by sub-groups such as the homeless.

Introduction

My purpose here is to consider what official data sources can contribute to the task of defining mental health care needs. I am going to begin by sketching out some features of the official data sources available. This will demonstrate some limitations and problems in using the data for this type of purpose. Finally I will propose some approaches which may, despite the problems, prove illuminating.

Official Data Sources

I should say at the outset what I mean by an official data source. Under this rubric I have included only data which some government agency requires to be collected in a relatively uniform way across the whole of England. Thus I have included hospital activity data and census data, and have excluded psychiatric case register data and special additional fields in individual district or regional PAS systems–informative though these might be–because they are not universally available. The other requirement I have made is that data sources should produce specific values for geographical units down to district health authorities. This unfortunately excludes other interesting data such as Home Office data relating to mentally abnormal offenders and the Mental Health Act Commission's statistics about compulsory treatment. While these provide interesting evidence of time trends, they are not published in a form which gives specific values for individual districts.

In any type of investigation it is normal to start by looking at such official data sources. The first reason for this is that they are readily available without additional cost of data collection. The second is that they allow comparisons to be made between one's own and other districts. With the computerised Performance Indicators which have been available in the last few years, it is possible to make comparisons with *similar* districts. A ready yard stick is thus available.

Mental Health Data

Official data sources that tell us about mental health can be divided into those relating to mental health services and those relating to other sources. Those relating to mental health services directly can again be divided into those which map out what services are there to be used, how many beds, how many CPNs, how many psychiatrists, etc. Then there are sources telling us how many people use the services and with what types of problem. Finally there is operational data about how the facilities are functioning, eg bed occupancy and throughput data.

Needs assessment based only upon service data is clearly not altogether satisfactory. Judging the volume of services needed from the volume of services used is inherently circular. Thus attempts have been made to find some external corroborative sources. Within the domain of official data sources two types of data exist. Direct evidence about the prevalence of psychiatric disorders comes from mortality data relating to suicide and alcohol-related disease such as cirrhosis of the liver. Indirect data is adduced from proxy measures of population deprivation levels. Recently Hirsch (1987), for the Royal College of Psychiatrists, has published a report arguing for the use of Jarman indices as a proxy measure of need for psychiatric services. Jarman has shown that there is a close relationship between deprivation level and admission rate.

Coverage of psychiatric service statistics

Let us consider for a moment what services are covered by current official statistics. Predictably, perhaps official data is strongest in the area of hospitals. The old Mental Health Enquiry and midnight bed state returns, superseded by the Korner in-patient data, give a lot of information about patients using beds. Much data is patient-based, rich in some types of detail and, as we shall see later, to some extent patient-linkable. Day care and hospital out-patient facilities are covered at the level of numbers of sessions, cases and new cases. Moving further away from the hospital, CPN case loads are covered in terms of numbers of visits, new cases, referral sources etc., but no linkage to the hospital data is possible. Thus it is not possible to establish how many people are receiving some service.

Services less similar to the routine medical style are less well covered. Thus Community Mental Health Centres are treated as day hospitals, attendances to see a consultant, or for groups of any kind etc. being indistinguishable. In some areas the shortcomings are clearly recognised. For example, clinical psychologists have argued that simply recording face-to-face clinical work underestimates their workload, which also includes support and consultancy work to many other staff. As a result, data about the percentage of overall time spent in patient contact is being requested. Time spent by consultants in advising GPs in their health centres would similarly not be apparent.

Some problems

The question we are attempting to ask is how much can we learn from such data about the extent of mental health problems in a district from the amount of treatment that happens?

Thus the first thing we should note is that the scope of official data sources does not include all the relevant facilities. This incompleteness potentially produces a serious source of bias. It is apparent that a district having what one might term an 'old-fashioned' mental health service, ie one heavily dependent on mental hospital beds and conventional hospital out-patient clinics and with access to longstay psychiatric beds for the care of long term mentally ill people, will be more completely documented than what one might term a 'modern' service with a community mental health centre, primary care level work by consultants and with residential and day care facilities for long-term patients in the voluntary sector.

There are two levels of this bias. The first is within health service facilities, so that the work of out patient clinics is reasonably well documented whilst that of community health centres is not. The second bias arises from the distribution of tasks between the health service and the voluntary sector. Current policy initiatives are shifting much of the work of caring for chronically mentally ill people away from the health service and towards the local authority and the voluntary sector. Data about local authority services is far less detailed than health service data, though with the requirement to produce annual community care reports this should improve. Voluntary sector services are not covered in any official statistics. Thus the use of official data to make cross district comparisons will only work between districts with broadly comparable service structures. Of course, it will be argued, people know what local authority and voluntary sector services are available in their own district. The problem however lies in using official data as a yardstick. Does the aggregate of all other services make a sensible comparison?

The second major problem with official service data is its poor quality and its incompleteness. There have been extensive teething problems with the implementation of Korner data sets in psychiatry. Many relevant areas such as community psychiatric nurses work were previously largely unrecorded. Data relating to events which take place in scattered locations is always much more difficult to capture than data relating to activity in big centres like hospitals. But for psychiatry even data regarding hospital functions has proved problematic. Under the old system, the Mental Health Enquiry, hospitals would fill in forms which were submitted to DHSS for central coding clerks to computerize. The new requirement is that the data should be submitted already coded on computer tapes. Unlike general hospitals, many of which already had computerized patient administration systems and most of which were developing them at the time of Korner implementation, many mental hospitals had not begun this process.

As a result, the first year of Korner mental health data (1987/8) has been considered so incomplete and unreliable that DoH figures will not be published until further years comparative data are available. A number of regional information specialists believe the hospital figures for that year are seriously flawed, even though hospital figures in general are better than the community figures.

At the next level, the completeness within the data sets, there have always been problems relating to mental hospital data. One reason is that unlike conventional acute hospital work it is common for a patient's stay to span more than one data year. In this case, incomplete records need to be filed in the admission year and then, hopefully linked at discharge with the remaining data for the episode. This linkage in the days of the Mental Health Enquiry was far from perfect. Another reason must be the level of commitment of staff involved. A couple of years ago I was asked if I could make a case for increasing the proportion of Mental Health resources in Mersey Region allocated to Liverpool on the basis of Mental Health Enquiry data. In the first available year of data there were a strikingly high proportion of patients homeless. Half way through the second year the homeless fraction dropped to well below the rate for the rest of the region and the 'missing data' code started to become frequent. I conclude there had been a change of staff.

The final major problem in using the data is the question of the presence or absence of the big mental hospital. In terms of quantitative data about activity this single factor can override almost anything. For bed provision, all the indicators of bed use are completely out of line with realistic expectations. Hampstead HA, for example, with Friern Hospital, shows about 8 beds per 1,000 population, with a throughput of 1.05 patients per bed per year. Districts dependant on a neighbouring HA for in-patient services show a complementary sort of distortion.

Some approaches

I have spent much time focusing on the difficulties of using official data sets to inform about public mental health and the needs for an adequacy of mental health services. I do not wish however to sound altogether nihilistic. John Yates (1982) has made the point that for all of their imperfections, official data sources can provide valuable insights if used with discrimination and this is certainly true for mental health services. There are two approaches to analysing official data which may be useful. The first is the use of multiple sources to provide an internal 'commentary'; the second is the isolation of specific groups.

Internal commentaries

What can official statistics show about how adequate the current service levels are to the needs of the local population?

Clearly this cannot be discerned simply from a district's position in the league table of eg beds per thousand population. However, more detailed patterns, built up from a number of indices can illuminate this. Occupancy levels are particularly useful. If an appropriate size for an acute unit is that size which will allow acute admissions to occur when necessary, then the occupancy rate must be a measure of adequacy since it is roughly possible to estimate the frequency with which admissions will fail for lack of a bed. There is no single appropriate level, for this will vary from district to district in relation to the total size of the bed stock and the frequency of emergency admissions. Nonetheless, appropriate occupany levels will usually be somewhere in the 80%s. In a letter to the BMJ, Hollander et al (1990) recorded inner London bed occupancies at around 97%. If correct, this is incompatible with adequate acute psychiatry. However, beds may be full because of inefficient use of services or because of blockage further down the stream. A high occupancy simply indicates that some feature of the in-patient service is not equal to the demands of local morbidity. While bed occupancy did not figure in the first set of Korner statistics, it was added to the data requirements in the year 1989/90.

The issue can be further illuminated by detailed analysis of stay lengths, and by throughput data and Jarman indices and needs to be considered in the light of the proportion of the bed stock which is for acute services.

The homeless – a special group

Finally I wish to look at how special need groups can be discerned from official statistics for a wide area. District statisticians can then identify how far those groups are represented in their own population as a measure of specific additional need. This can be illustrated by looking at homelessness.

This approach requires analysis of the official data sets collected in ways which are not at present undertaken by the Department. With increasingly powerful small computers the approach is possible. I want to show you some results of an analysis I undertook using Mental Health Enquiry raw data to map the 'careers' of individual patients over a nine year period from 1976–84. The original raw data tapes sent by the then DHSS to regional health authorities permitted this. By separating out data for individual hospitals and then combining the annual files for each hospital it was possible to identify recurring instances of the same hospital unit

Figure 1
Average annual bed use in years following first admission, by residence at time of first admission

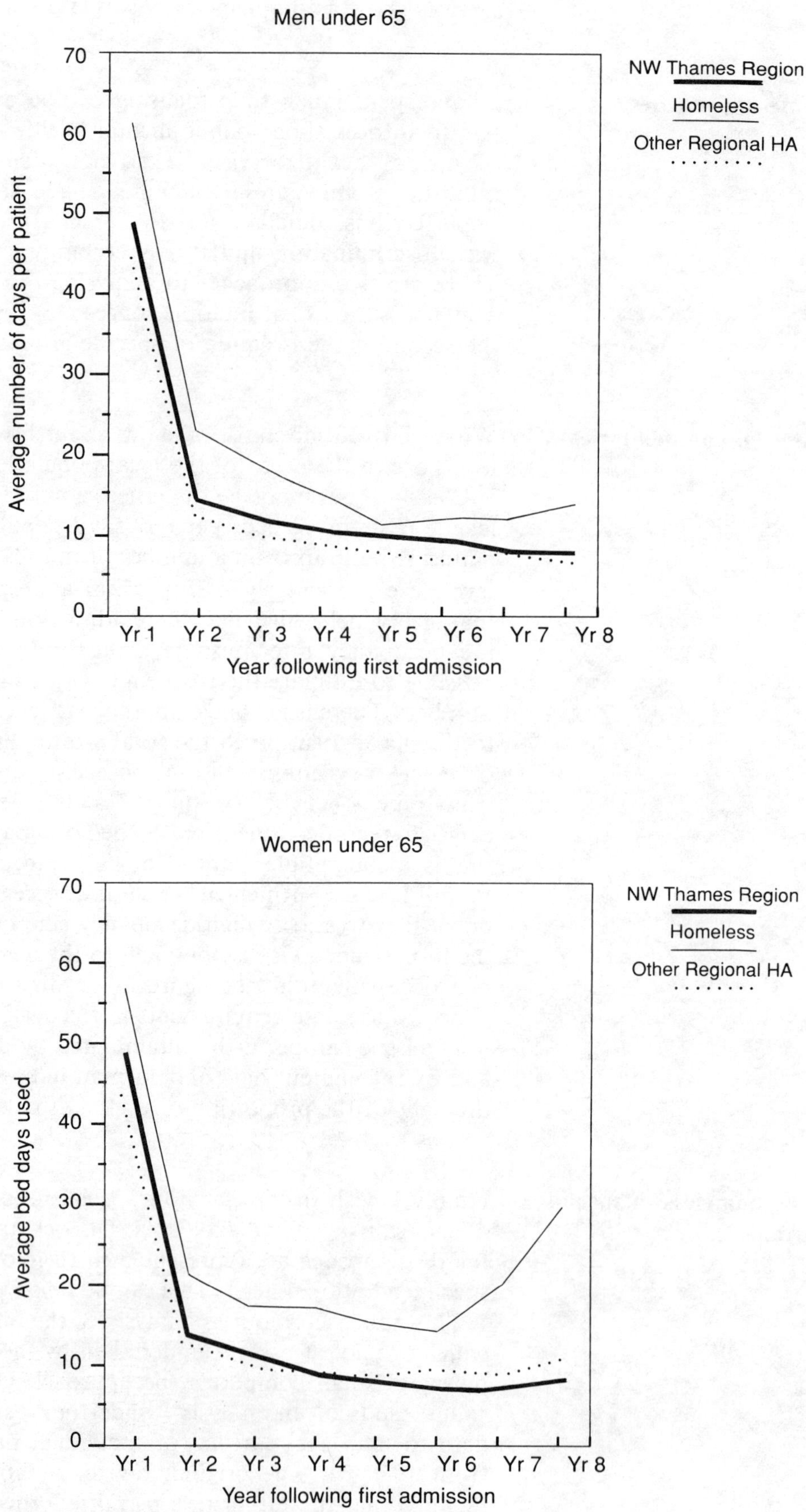

Figure 2
Proportion of first admission patients homeless or in temporary lodgings NW Thames Region hospitals, 1976–84

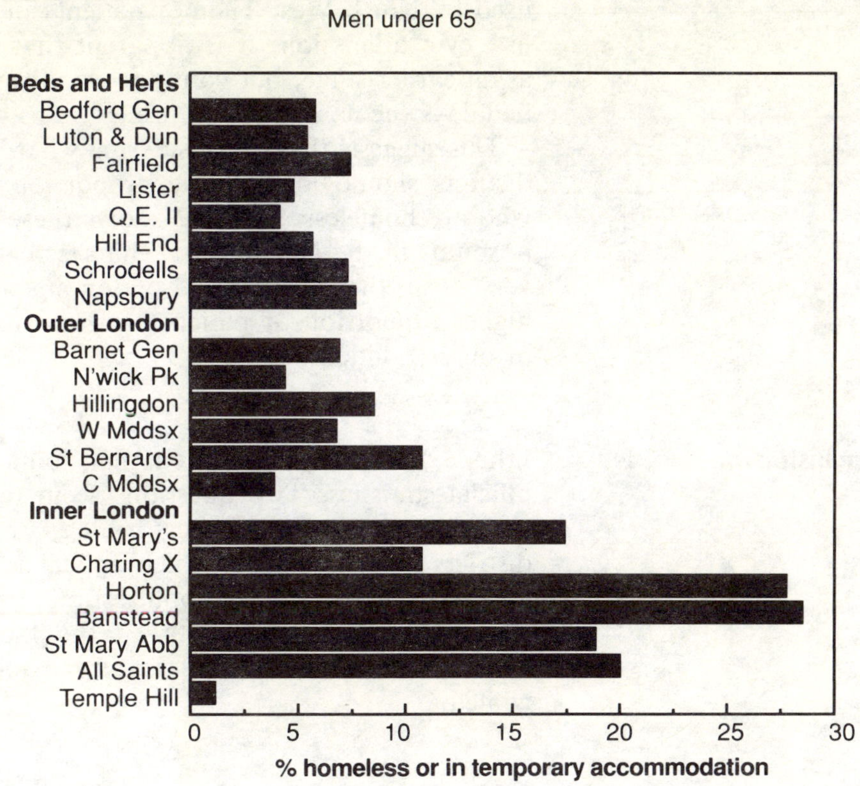

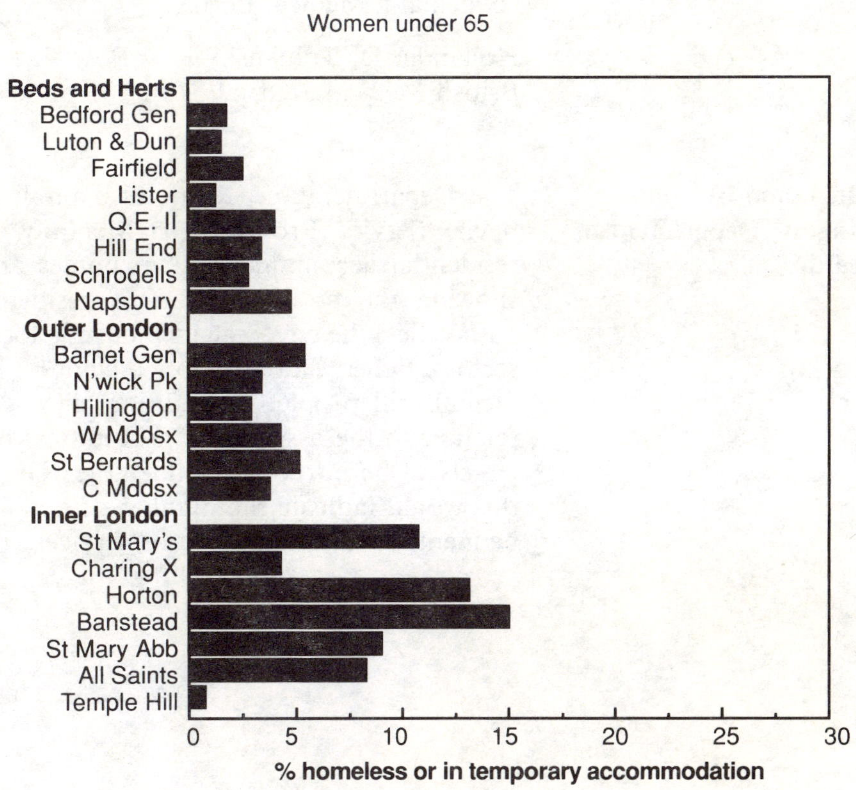

number, sex and date of birth. This gave a reasonably satisfactory method of linking the successive admissions of individuals. Individuals were classified as homeless or not on the basis of the place of residence code in the first admission record. Figure 1 shows the average number of bed days used by North-West Thames patients in each 12 month period after their first ever admission. It is apparent that homeless people do not drop out at an earlier stage, but continue steadily to use about twice the number of bed days the non-homeless use.

This suggests that in considering what is an appropriate level of facilities, districts should look at the proportion of their newly admitted patients who are homeless. Figure 2 shows these proportions for all of the mental hospitals in the North-West Thames region at the time of the study. It is very clear that the inner London mental hospitals have a substantially higher proportion of patients with no fixed abode than hospitals in rural or outer London.

Conclusion

I hope I have demonstrated that some useful lessons can come out of official statistics. Two questions seem to be addressable: how adequately are a district's services performing; how much of a representation do districts have of groups which appear to have special needs? It would be unwise to be too precise about estimations from this source, and it is vital to be able to take account of the facilities in the social services and voluntary sectors. Nonetheless, with careful analysis, useful insights can be gained.

References

Hirsch, S R (1988) 'Psychiatric Beds and Resources, Factors Influencing Bed Use and Service Planning'. Gaskell Imprint, Royal College of Psychiatrists.

Yates, J (1982) 'Hospital Beds: A Problem for Diagnosis and Management.' Heinemann Medical Books.

Hollander D, Tohiansky R & Powell, R (1990) 'Crisis in Admission Beds' British Medical Journal, Vol. 301 p. 664.

Addendum by John Lithgow, Department of Health

The Department of Health also publishes official statistics on 'Personal Social Service Provision to Mentally Ill People'. This covers data on residential accommodation in homes and hostels for mentally ill people, showing the total numbers of residents and those supported by local authorities; the coverage includes the local authority, voluntary and private sectors. Other data available includes numbers of places in day centres for mentally ill people. In addition, new collections are being considered in relation to the assessment procedures to be carried out by local authority panels to be introduced under the NHS and Community Care Act 1990: this would indicate the number of people assessed who were considered to be mentally ill and in need of services.

How Can we Measure Mental Health?

Dr Alastair Macdonald

Abstract

In this presentation I shall be making certain assumptions and taking certain liberties with language. I assume that mental health is inverse of mental ill-health, and that mental ill-health has three distinguishable components – mental illness, mental disorder and mental distress.

Mental distress is the unpleasant subjective experience of mental ill-health.

Mental disorder is impairment of functioning (of self or others) cause by mental ill-health.

Mental illness is attributed to those with mental ill-health when the features of the ill-health conform to a recognisable pattern; this pattern is distinguished from others by its name – the diagnosis.

We can measure all three. In individuals we might wish to monitor response to treatment, for instance, but this is unusual. Far more common is measurement in groups usually asking two sorts of questions:

(i) *how many?* implying categorisation. How many people in a population would attract diagnoses by a psychiatrist, and what diagnoses? This requires the use of standardised psychiatric interviews, now often subject to algorithmic analysis using rules devised by leading psychiatrists. I will discuss the notions of reliability and validity. The interviews may have to be preceded by a self-completed questionnaire – the '2-stage screening' process. The approximate nature of these procedures confine their utility to groups; I distinguish them from screening for individuals with mental illness, eg in general practice.

(ii) *how bad?* implying dimensionality. It is usual to express distress and disorder as dimensions. I will mention depression symptom scales, the GHQ, and others. They must be sensitive to change for intervention/ outcome studies. Some can be used with cut-points to mimic categorical judgements.

I will conclude by pointing out the high levels of agreement about prevalence in various settings, and the importance of measurement in assessing advances, and clearing away the dead wood of irrelevant procedures.

Introduction

I'm not going to answer the question 'Why should we measure mental health?' I hope that will be obvious. Also, I have no intention of churning out a catalogue of rating scales and techniques to be used. Instead, I will sketch an outline of the current basis of psychiatric epidemiology, the process of direct measurement in groups and populations. But first, a word about language.

Those non-psychiatrists among you will often be baffled by the language that psychiatrists use. Psychiatrists themselves are, if anything, more baffled; but also annoyed, mainly because they cannot communicate easily with each other, and also because they cannot make themselves understood to anyone else either. To answer the question posed by the title of my talk I shall take gross liberties with the language of psychiatry. I do this to produce an illusion of clarity (which, of course, is spurious). I realise that I shall thus annoy further those who have spent a lot of time thinking and reading about these things, but time is short!

Components of mental ill-health

For this talk I assume that mental health is the inverse of mental ill-health, so measurement of ill-health will do. (I realise that I part with the WHO[1] here). Next, I assume that mental ill-health has 3 distinguishable components: mental distress, mental disorder and mental illness. All these are measurable.

Mental distress is the unpleasant subjective experience of mental ill-health. For instance, the pain of a bleak depression, said by many to be worse than so-called 'physical' pain. The distress is not necessarily confined, of course, to the person with ill-health.

Mental disorder is impairment of *functioning* related to mental ill-health. Again, this impairment can be in the sufferer (eg failure to cope with work, or taking the 'sick role') or impairment in the functioning of *others*, (eg in carers of those with chronic schizophrenia).

It is arguable that there can be no isolated dysfunction or distress in an individual, except on a desert island. These are the arguments against what Jonathan Miller calls 'morbid individualism'. It is quite possible for the bulk of the distress or disorder to occur in those *other* than the person with mental ill-health, eg in certain disorders of personality.

Mental illness is attributed to those with mental ill-health when the features of the ill-health (pattern of symptoms, signs, course, family and past history) conform to a recognisable pattern; this pattern is distinguished from others by its name–a *diagnosis*. The diagnosis is short-hand for a hypothesis about how the ill-health arose, why it takes the form it does, what biochemical abnormalities there may be (if any), and what will happen to the person with ill-health (a) if nothing is done and (b) if some intervention is carried out. The attribution of a diagnosis is thus a *categorical* process. Either the diagnostic hypothesis is attributed to a person or it is not. Furthermore, the attribution is obviously most useful when it is made by someone with wide experience of possible hypotheses, in other words, *psychiatrists* should make diagnoses.

I must point out that there is a similarly categorical question at the level above–a question that has provoked a lot of discussion in psychiatric epidemiology–namely 'Is he/she mentally ill at all?' (Another variant is 'Is he/she a 'case' of mental illness?') It is easy to answer 'yes' when the pattern of symptoms forms a recognisable pattern, ie a psychiatrist has already attributed a specific diagnostic hypothesis. It is *not* easy when there are symptoms or signs but they form no recognisable pattern. In that case we are often guided by whether or not there is associated distress and/or disorder. Whilst it is clearly important for it to be *psychiatrists* who say 'I cannot attribute any specific diagnostic hypothesis to this person', it is not obvious why psychiatrists are any better than anyone else at saying whether or not that particular person is a 'case'. So, in my view, the lay attribution of 'caseness' is quite appropriate–'Private Eye' is free to decide that Saddam Hussein is a 'case' (not because he invaded Kuwait, not by threatening to plunge the whole region, perhaps the whole world, into a dreadful war, but because he suggested that Margaret Thatcher was irresponsible). But it is inappropriate for 'Private Eye' to say *what* diagnosis should be attributed to this man. Indeed, apart from saying he was 'stark, staring bonkers', they wisely refrained from any specific diagnosis.

I hope it is obvious from this rather windy introduction that the measurement of components of mental ill-health involve rather different principles.

I shall take measurement here as meaning the answering of two sorts of question – How many? and How bad?

How Many?

'How many people in this population are cases of mental illness?' I hope it is clear from what I have said that the most useful data is obtained not by asking this question at all. An answerable question is: 'How many people in this population would attract a specific diagnostic hypothesis, and which?'

I am not going to enter into all the methodological difficulties here, but simply state that the most common procedure is to administer, to a random sample of the population, a standardised psychiatric interview. In this, the sorts of question and order of question are heavily constrained, if not immutable, and the responses coded in a pre-determined way. Interviewers are specially trained in the use of the interview, but are not always psychiatrists.

Strictly speaking, attempts should be made to check that interviewers are using the interview in the same way as others in previous surveys and as each other (inter-rater reliability). This is rarely checked, and a convenient assumption is often made that the inter-rater reliability is, in some magic way, a function of the interview itself rather than the procedure of which the interview is a part, and, once measured and deemed satisfactory in one survey, is forgotten about.

The coded responses are then submitted to an analysis which produces diagnostic categories. In the past this was done using more or less complex arithmetic; increasingly this is done using rule-based computerised algorithms. Who writes the rules? The answer is: leading psychiatrists, attempting to enshrine their clinical practice in machine code. Professor John Wing is immortalised in the CATEGO program which analyses the Present State Examination interview[2]; Prof John Copeland in AGECAT, which does the same for the Geriatric Mental State schedule[3]. Much to everyone's disgust, these procedures seem to generate results that accord surprisingly well with most clinical psychiatrists, ie criterion validity seems quite high. Of course, unlike real psychiatrists, confronted with the same symptoms, these programs always produce the same diagnoses, so one source of variability is excluded. These procedures are quick enough to be carried out at the point of data collection: we can generate AGECAT diagnostic categories instantaneously by interviewing the patient with a lap-top computer rather than paper and pencil.

The main difficulty of these procedures is the expense of interviewing large numbers of people who turn out not to have any great pathology, especially if the procedure demands a psychiatric training for the interviewers. (This cost is the reason why interviews in which the interviewer made judgements about the subject's response, ie had to have professional training, are used less than those in which the subject's response is accepted without qualification). One way round this is to target the interviews on those from the population who show an increased risk of being diagnosable, by using some cheap and cheerful method of initial 'screening'. The most popular of such screening methods is to use a self-rated, perhaps postal, questionnaire which is essentially a symptom counter, ie. dimensional, and select a cut-point above which the full interview is carried out. This is the 'two-stage screening' method of psychiatric epidemiology. An example of a pairing of a screening questionnaire with a standard interview is the General Health Questionnaire and the Clinical Interview Schedule combination[4]. Selecting an appropriate cut-point is problematic and to back-calculate from the results of the interview you need to know just how sensitive and specific the screening questionnaire is. This sort of screening introduces error into a procedure and emphasises the fact that the most you will get out of any survey is an *estimate* in the population. Again it is surprising how alike estimates in similar populations are.

I want to emphasise the 'two-stage screening' procedure is an epidemiological cost-cutting exercise for making estimates in *groups*, and has nothing whatever to do with 'screening' for *individuals* with disorder, for instance the screening for dementia and depression in 75 year old patients by GPs.

How bad?

I think that psychiatric epidemiology has licked the basic problem of 'How many?' questions, apart from minor difficulties with 'caseness' and diagnostic categories. There are reasonably well-accepted procedures for estimating the prevalence of all major psychiatric diseases with acceptable accuracy and economy in most populations (community samples, attenders in general practice and out-patients, acute in-patients and long-stay patients).

But we still have a long way to go in the quantification of distress and disorder associated with mental ill-health. This is important for two main purposes.

First, in the comparison of levels of distress and disorder in two groups, such as in the assessment of distress in the carers of dementia sufferers compared with the age/sex-matched general population or control group. The finding of consistently higher scale scores (on the General Health Questionnaire, here used as a dimensional scale) confirms the need for interventions to reduce the distress and disability caused by dementia in the community[5]. The use of diagnostic ('how many?') procedures would certainly reveal little, since prevalence of diagnostic categories is low enough, even in this highly stressed group, to demand unreasonably large samples.

Second, such quantification is vital in order to carry out reasonable studies of intervention or service delivery and in this case, to assess eg whether respite care reduces GHQ scores in carers. There are certainly hundreds, and probably thousands of dimensional scales (as interviews or self-rated questionnaires) that purport to quantify every dimension of psychological functioning and associated distress, yet very few indeed are subject to the intense development and thought that applied to the diagnostic procedures I have been discussing earlier.What are *really* needed now are scales that are designed to be sensitive to change. This means that they must have the following properties: their validity must be respectable (the degree with which they measure what they say they measure); their potential inter-rater reliability must be high; their potential test-retest reliability must be high; and, most important, their validity as *change measures* must be checked against other indices of change. The development of such scales represents an enormous investment, and many may balk at the cost.

Conclusion

What of the future? I hope we will see the development of more change-sensitive scales for distress and disorder; I am sure that we will see more scales. (Those who declare a moratorium on scale development always do so just after they publish theirs). I hope we will see the use of portable computers to speed up data-collection and improve accuracy; I am sure we will see more personalised algorithms and also computer-administered interviews like IPSAG (the Clinical Interview Schedule in micro form[6]). These are a sort of hybrid between cheap self-rating questionnaires and costly research interviews. I have said nothing about measurement in clinical settings, for the purposes of assessing individual diagnoses and changes in distress and disorder. I hope that we will see rating scales that will place our clinical management[7] and individual screening on a firmer basis than at present. Generally speaking, I am sure that we will see more rating scales.

Appendix – A random sample of scales

Montgomery-Asberg Depression Rating Scale
Hamilton Depression Rating Scale
Brief Psychiatric Rating Scale
Blessed Dementia Rating Scale
Comprehensive Psychopathology Scale
Global Assessment Scale
Bech-Rafaelson Melancholia Scale
Rating for Emotional Blunting
Scale for the Assessment of Negative Symptoms
Depression and OBS scales of the CARE
Mini-mental status examination
Newcastle Rating Scale for Depression
Hoehn & Yahr disability scale
Katz ADL scale
State-trait anxiety inventory
Tellegen Absorption Scale
Harvard Group Scale of Hypnotic susceptibility
Spielberger state-trait Anxiety Inventory
Automatic thoughts questionnaire

References (1978)

1. WHO 'Health for all by the year 2000'.
2. Wing, J K, Cooper, J E, Sartorius, N (1974) The description and classification of psychiatric symptoms: an instruction manual for the Present State Examination and CATEGO system. Cambridge University Press, London.
3. Copeland, J R M et al (1987) Using the GMS-AGECAT package. British Journal of Psychiatry 150, 815–823.
4. Goldberg, D P, Blackwell, B (1970) Psychiatric illness in general practice: a detailed study using a new method of case identification. British Medical Journal 2, 429–443.
5. Gilleard, C J (1987) Influence of emotional distress among supporters on the outcome of psychogeriatric day care. British Journal of Psychiatry 150, 219–223
6. Lewis, G, Pelosi, A J, Glover, E, Wilkinson, G, Stansfield, S A, Williams, P, Shepherd, M (1988) the development of a computerised assessment for minor psychiatric disorder. Psychological Medicine 18, 737–745.
7. Hiller, W, Zaudig, M, Mobour, W (1990) Development of diagnostic checklists for use in routine clinical care. Archives of General Psychiatry, 47, 782–784.

Filters to Care–A Model

Professor David Goldberg

Abstract

This paper describes four filters which stand between people in the community and in-patient facilities for the mentally ill: illness behaviour, ability to detect disorder by care-givers, willingness to refer mentally disordered patients to specialist services, and admission behaviour by mental health professionals.

The first part of the paper summarises research relevant to the filters in the past ten years, and gives revised estimates for morbidity at each level in order to estimate the permeability of each filter. It is concluded that although the third filter (referral behaviour) is more permeable than previous estimates had suggested, it is still the least permeable of the four. Activities of mental health professionals in primary care settings can be thought of as direct onslaughts upon the third filter.

In the second part of the paper we consider three possible ways of considering the mental health needs of a population: the prevalence of disorder in that population; the extent to which the needs of those with common mental disorders are being met; and the extent to which the needs of those with more severe kinds of mental disorders are being met. Each of these can be addressed in a number of ways. We argue that estimates of the period prevalence of disorder among attenders is a reasonable proxy for the first problem; that combined studies of the second and third filter are ways of addressing the second; but that statistics from the mental health service must be used to address the third.

Introduction

In order to be seen by the mental illness services, an individual must seek care (or help must be sought by someone on his behalf); a mental disorder must be detected by a care-giver; and the care-giver must refer to the specialist services. Finally, in order to achieve the status of an in-patient and thus enter official statistical tables, the patient must be admitted to hospital by a mental health professional. These four filters can be thought of as (1) illness behaviour; (2) the detection of disorder; (3) referral behaviour and (4) admission behaviour.

This framework was suggested by Goldberg and Huxley (1980), and served to organise epidemiological data about mental illness into groupings which depended upon how far along the pathway individuals had reached. Approximately two-thirds of patients who are eventually seen by specialist mental health services come directly from primary care settings, with a further quarter coming from medical clinics and emergency rooms in hospitals (Gater et al 1991). The filters were thought of as being between five levels at which survey data could be considered, each one corresponding to a stage on the pathway to psychiatric care. It is clear that a filter that holds many people back is more important than one which lets most people through, and our original figures showed that the 2nd and 3rd filters let the fewest people through, with the 3rd filter being the least permeable of all. Goldberg and Huxley (1991) have recalculated these levels and their most recent estimates are shown as Table 1.

Table 1 Mental illness in hospital and community settings: Data from Greater Manchester during 1982/1983

Annual period prevalences per 1,000 population at risk [unduplicated counts]	
Mental Disorders in the community	250–315
Mental Disorders among GP attenders	230
Mental disorders recognised by GP[1]	101.5
Mental disorders treated by MI services[2]	20.8
Mental admissions to hospital[2]	3.3

[1] these data are for England, 1982, from the 3rd National Morbidity Survey
[2] data from Salford Case Register, 1983

At levels 1 and 2 the estimates are based on responses to the General Health Questionnaire (Goldberg & Williams 1988), and correspond to a severity or disorder equivalent to a 'case' as defined by the DSM-3 Classification of the American Psychiatric Association, or by the Clinical Interview Schedule, or by the 'ID4' level of Wing's 'Index of Definition' (Wing and others 1977).

Somewhat lower levels would be obtained by using the level of severity more often associated with psychiatric out-patients, the ID5 level. However, the lower level has been preferred because it corresponds to concepts of caseness thought appropriate by workers in primary care settings, and the model itself heavily depends upon events in general medical settings.

The estimated period prevalence in the community is perhaps the most controversial figure shown above, which is based upon an estimated point prevalence of minor disorder of 18% in South Manchester, and recent surveys which have compared annual inceptions to point prevalence for both anxiety disorders and depressive illness. Repeated estimates at level 2 by our Unit over the past 12 years give no grounds for supposing that estimated prevalence is changing with time, although there are some increases at level 4 and 5. For example, between 1983 and 1989 the level 4 prevalence in Salford increased from 20.9 to 23.5/1,000, while the level 5 levels changed from 3.3 to 5.7/1,000.

The First Filter: Illness Behaviour

Williams and others (1990) have argued that almost all of the variance of illness behaviour is explained by the severity of the problem, propensity to seek help, accessibility of services and the availability of alternatives. Of these, illness-related problems are easily the most important. Distress as measured by the GHQ accounts for about 20% of the variance of all medical consultations, and there is a direct, linear relationship between GHQ score and the probability of consultation. Sex has an independent, additive effect upon the probability of consulting, and there is some evidence that consultations on behalf of others largely accounts for the increased female rates. Other factors that exert an independent, additive effect upon consultations include self-assessed health status, the presence of chronic disease, and unemployment in males (Williams and others 1986).

It is possible that the earlier estimates of period prevalence for common disorders in the community were too low, and these rates have been revised upwards in the light of three recent studies relating to inception rates of anxiety and depressive disorders. Thus, it is probable that the unmet need of those who do not consult was under-estimated. To the extent that treatable illnesses exist in the population not seeking care, they probably consist of depressive disorders and agoraphobics, and the public health implications consist of better health education and the ready availability of mental health care in community settings.

The Second Filter: The Detection of Disorder

The ability of GPs to identify mental disorders is highly variable, but all subsequent surveys agree with our earlier estimate that a substantial proportion of mental disorders are not detected. Those with superior interview skills, good previous knowledge of their patient, and favourable attitudes towards psychological disorder are better able to detect disorder, and the ability can be modified by training.

Failure to detect disorder can be thought of as a collusive non-event by doctor and patient, each determined to confine the medical encounter to the exclusion of a physical disease as a cause for the patient's symptoms. The available evidence suggests that feedback of the results of screening questionnaires is only worthwhile if doctors have received prior assistance in how to manage disorder, but there is convergent evidence that detected depressive illnesses have a better outcome than missed illnesses. However, it should be appreciated that a substantial group of disorders that do not pass the second filter are self-limiting disorders which would remit without medical intervention.

The public health implications of this work are two-fold: more work needs to be done in providing training courses for GPs in training, and further research on patients should be focused on groups where detection promises some definite return–either in terms of a better clinical outcome, or by reducing the costs of unnecessary physical investigations.

The Third Filter: Referral to Specialist Services

It must be appreciated that disorders referred to mental health services are very much more severe than those not referred, both in terms of their 'index of definition' and their clinical diagnosis. Inspection of the diagnosis-specific annual period prevalences at levels 3 and 4 reveal that adjustment disorders and anxiety states are least likely to be referred, while the majority of cases of schizophrenia and organic states are sent on. Indeed, the figures for schizophrenia are higher at level 4 than at level 3.

There is incontrovertible evidence that men are preferentially referred for specialist help (Goldberg & Huxley 1991): indeed, one study in Edinburgh has shown that for every 100 women in the community with a diagnosis, only 3 are known to the mental illness service (Sashidharan et al 1988). Women below the age of 35 are particularly unlikely to be referred. It is of interest that the divorced, separated and widowed are less likely to be referred, since if anything they pass the first two filters more easily than others.

In public health terms, service developments with direct access by mental health professionals in primary care settings are of crucial importance in allowing interventions to reach a wider range of patients. However, at present such services are uncoordinated and poorly managed, and it is likely that a very much more efficient use could be made of available manpower if management was introduced at this level. The old multi-disciplinary team, hospital based and medically dominated, has vanished from many parts of the country. The 'managed multi-disciplinary team', available to patients in both hospital and community, should take its place.

The Fourth Filter: Admission to Hospital Beds

Those admitted to psychiatric beds continue to be very much more severely ill than those seen in out-patients. Well over half of the disorders admitted to beds are rare in community settings. Admissions are rising in Salford despite increasing provision of community services; the filter becomes more permeable for the elderly. As beds are closed mean duration of stay is dropping in the face of sustained admission rates. The suicidal and the homicidal pass this filter readily, and it is also likely that lack of social support is an important variable.

From a public health standpoint it is necessary to monitor mean duration of stay in a context of re-admission rates, since it is important that patients are not discharged before they are able to manage in the community. The 'Care in the Community' recommendations mean that it is desirable for those responsible for providing care to set up and maintain a register of those thought to require joint care by health and social services, and such registers should provide an important indicator of perceived needs of the most vulnerable, as well as the extent to which these needs have been met.

Indicators of Need

One can ask three kinds of question about the mental health needs in a particular district:

1. what is the prevalence of common mental disorders?

2. to what extent are the needs of those with common disorders being met by the local services?

3. to what extent are the needs of those with severe mental disorders being met by the service?

Each of these questions can be addressed in a number of ways, depending upon the information which is locally available.

The Prevalence of Common Disorders

i. It should be appreciated that common mental disorders are more frequent in areas of high social deprivation, so that those responsible for preparing reports should make themselves aware of characteristics which can be derived from Census Data about their own district. An example of such a global measure would be Jarman (1983) underprivileged area score [UPA score]. Jarman and his colleagues (1990) have shown that the UPA score for DHAs correlates +0.82 with actual psychiatric admissions. A still better correlation, of +0.87, can be found between actual admissions and three other variables: the % of illegitimate births, the number of 1st notifications for drug dependence, and the standardised mortality ratio for that health district. It is not suggested that these are in any sense causal variables, but they are social indicators of need for service. Areas within a Health District which are known to be particularly socially disadvantaged should be targeted for special study.

ii. Surveys of random samples of the population are a direct way of addressing the problem, but they are very expensive to mount.

iii. An acceptable, and much easier, alternative is to study prevalence of disorders among those seeking care. If there were substantial numbers of mental disorders responsive to an available treatment among those who never sought care this would be unreasonable, but the available evidence suggests that most of such patients do attend their general practitioner, although they are often presenting physical complaints. For this purpose consecutive attenders in primary care clinics are screened for a fixed period of time using a screening questionnaire of know validity.

The probable prevalence of disorders among consecutive attenders is then obtained using a formula suggested by Diamond and Lilienfeld (1963):

$$(\% \text{ high scores} \times \text{PPV}) + (\% \text{ low scorers} \times \{1\text{-NPV}\})$$

PPV = Positive predictive value
NPV = Negative predictive value
[For example, in British General Practice the GHQ-28 with a threshold of 4/5 has a PPV of 63.6% and a NPV of 92.2% for DSM-3 caseness].

Provided that this estimate is based upon a sufficiently large, representative sample, and one knows the proportion of a given population that consult their family doctor in the course of one year, then the estimated annual prevalence in the population is given by

(estimated prevalence among attenders) × (proportion consulting, annual)

Example:

During a study on a large housing estate in South Manchester the General Health Questionnaire was administered to 1,528 patients attending their family doctors for treatment. It was found that 51% of them had high scores on the screening questionnaire, which meant that, had they been interviewed by a doctor using DSM-3 research criteria for diagnosis, that 36% would have been found to be suffering from a mental disorder [mainly anxiety disorders and depressive disorders].

Since it is known that 71% of this population consulted their family doctors in the course of the year, we may calculate that the annual period prevalence of mental disorder among attenders at primary care is 257/1,000 at risk/year.

The extent to which needs are being met

Once more, there are various ways of addressing this problem.

i. The ability to detect mental disorders can be assessed by asking general practitioners to make their own assessments of patients who have completed a screening questionnaire. Doctors are selected who are representative of a district or an area within that district, and each completes a special rating form for a run of 100 consecutive patients.[1] This form asks for information about all patients within that run of 100 who were thought to suffer from a mental disorder: the doctor has to code the diagnosis, and to give brief details of treatment. The detection skills of the doctors can be assessed by expressing the proportion of the high scorers identified as cases to the predicted prevalence in that practice [the 'identification index']. In South Manchester, the average identification index for a family doctor is 60%, which compares favourably with earlier figures for 91 doctors in Greater Manchester.

ii. The extent to which disorders are being treated can be derived from the form, and it is of interest to examine the proportion of all those identified as cases who receive treatment. These figures can be converted to period prevalences, for comparison with the figures mentioned earlier.

Example:

28% of 2,200 patients rated by 22 doctors on the Wythenshawe Estate were diagnosed by them as suffering from a mental disorder. Using the earlier argument about consultation rate, we may therefore calculate that the annual period prevalence of mental disorders recognised by family doctors is 196/1,000/year.

---

[1] The '100 Patient Form' is available from the Mental Illness Research Unit, University of Manchester.

Not all disorders recognised by family doctors are thought to need medical treatment. Treatment–either counselling or medication–was recorded for 89% of those receiving a label of mental illness from their family doctor. This represents a treated prevalence of 175/1,000 population at risk/year.

iii. The extent to which identified patients are treated by the specialist mental health services is another way of examining the third filter. This can be examined in three different ways. If specialist mental health staff working in the community are prepared to give an account of their clinical work a direct assessment can be made of the extent to which various disorders are being treated. Unfortunately those working in the community are not always prepared to say what is wrong with their patients, saying that 'diagnosis is a matter for doctors'. In default of such information, the permeability of the filter can be assessed in two ways–by examining the GPs returns on the '100 patients' forms to see how many were referred on for help, and by comparing morbidity at level 3 of the model with morbidity at level 4.

Example:

During the survey year, 341 patients were referred, or managed to get seen by, the mental illness services practices with a combined list size of 20,934. This corresponds to an annual period prevalence of 16.3/1,000 at risk/year.

The needs of those with severe disorders

It is difficult to draw firm conclusions about the need for in-patient facilities from the actual numbers of beds available, although these should be recorded under three headings: short stay and long stay for those <65, and facilities for those >65.

i. For each of these, it is of interest to record % occupancy; mean duration of stay; and diagnosis specific re-admission rates. It is desirable that occupancy should be about 85%–any more than this suggests that there are insufficient beds to run the service properly. Other indicators of insufficiency are short durations of stay combined with high re-admission rates. However, these figures should be interpreted with caution, since it is desirable to tolerate some re-admissions if long stays in hospital can be avoided (see Goldberg & Jones, 1980). However, if short stays can only be achieved at the price of high re-admission rates for the functional psychoses, it suggests that all is not well.

ii. A good mental illness service should keep an 'at risk' register of vulnerable people thought to be in need of joint local authority/health authority care. This register should identify a named key worker who is responsible for each patient, and information should be available concerning the frequency with which patients on this register have contacts with the service. The numbers of those without a named key worker, the numbers of patients assigned to each key worker, and the number who have lost contact with the service are all potential indices of need.

The information given so far is summarised in Table 2, and can be compared with data for the Greater Manchester area given in Table 1.

In this example, it is gratifying to note that, despite the rather higher rate of disorder among attenders, that GPs working in the area display a high awareness of psychological problems, and provide some treatment for a high proportion of the disorders that they detect. A sub-study of a new

Table 2 Mental illness in hospital and community settings: Data for South Manchester DHA during 1989/1990

Annual period prevalences per 1,000 population at risk [unduplicated counts]	
Mental Disorders among GP attenders	257
Mental disorders recognised by GP	196
Mental disorders treated by GP	175
Mental disorders treated by MI services	12.6
Mental admissions to hospital	4.1

community mental illness team targeted on primary care showed that it was possible to more than double the rate at which patients were treated by specialist services (Jackson et al 1991).

References

Diamond, E and Lilienfeld, A (1962). Effects of errors in classification and diagnosis in various types of epidemiological studies. American Journal of Public Health, 52, 1,137–1,144.

Gater, R, de Almeida e Sousa, R, Caraveo, J, Chandrasekar, C, Dhadphale, M, Goldberg, D, al Kathiri, A, de Llano G, Mubbashar, M, Silhan K, Thong D, Torres, F, and Sartorius, N (1991). The Pathways to Psychiatric Care: A Cross cultural study. Psychological Medicine [in press].

Goldberg & Huxley (1980). Mental Illness in the Community. The Pathway to Psychiatric Care. London: Tavistock.

Goldberg & Huxley (1991). Common Mental Disorders: A Bio-social Model. London: Routledge.

Goldberg, D and Jones, R (1980). The Costs and Benefits of Psychiatric Care In The Social Consequences of Psychiatric Illness (E L Robins, P Clayton and J Wing) New York: Brunner/Mazel.

Goldberg, D and Williams, P. (1988) A User's Guide to the General Health Questionnaire. Windsor: NFER.

Jackson, M, Gater, R, Goldberg, D, Tantam, D, Taylor, H and Loftus, L (1991) A new community mental health team based in primary care: II Impact on service utilisation. [submitted to British Journal of Psychiatry].

Jarman, B (1983) Identification of underprivileged areas. British Medical Journal, 286, 1,705–1,709.

Jarman, B, White, P, Hirsch, S and Driscoll, R (1990) Factors affecting psychiatric admission rates in England. (personal communication).

Morbidity Statistics from General Practice. 3rd National Survey, 1981–1982. (1986) London: HMSO.

Sashidharan, S, Surtees, P, Kreitman, N, Ingham, J and Miller, P (1988). Hospital Treated and General Population Morbidity from Affective Disorders: Comparison of prevalence and Inception Rates. British Journal of Psychiatry, 152, 499–505.

Williams, P, Tarnopolsky, A, Hand, D, and Shepherd, M (1986). Minor psychiatric morbidity and general practice consultations: the West London Survey Psychological Medicine Monograph Supplements No. 9.

Williams, P, Wilkinson G, and Arreghini, E (1990). The Determinants of Help seeking for psychological disorders in primary care settings. In Psychological Disorders in General Medical Settings (ed. N Sartorius, D Goldberg, G de Girolamo, J Costa e Silva, Y LeCrubier and H-U Wittchen) Bern: Huber-Hogrefe.

Wing, J K (1989). Health Services Planning and Research. Contributions from psychiatric case registers. London: Gaskell.

Wing, J, Nixon, J, Mann, S and Leff, J (1977). Reliability of the PSE in a population survey. Psychological Medicine, 7, 505–516.

Applying a Model: Experiences from a District

Dr Alison Hill and Dr Ruaridh Milne

Abstract

Milton Keynes, the new city in the north of Buckinghamshire, has a population of about 190,000 at present, and a steady population growth of about 6,000 people per year. A community mental health team was established in Bletchley in 1986, the rest of the district is served by a less formal network of community psychiatric nurses and social workers, with psychiatrists working from the general hospital base.

Introduction

In our annual report this year on the health of the population we put a section on mental health. Here we will describe the beginnings of an approach to needs assessment, using local data. A major weakness of our report is the lack of comparative data, but we hope that the thinking we have been through will contribute to the process of developing valuable indicators of need.

Milton Keynes is a new city in the north of Buckinghamshire. Its population is about 190,000 at present, and it has a steady population growth of about 6,000 people per year. The county mental hospital is in Aylesbury, but is due to close in 1991. From the beginning, the emphasis in Milton Keynes has been on community mental health services, with relatively few hospital beds available. A community mental health team was established in Bletchley in 1986. The rest of the district is at present served by a less formal network of community psychiatric nurses and social workers, with psychiatrists working from the general hospital base, though it is intended that the remaining areas will ultimately be served by community mental health teams. Milton Keynes also has a very active MIND group which provides a large number projects and programmes.

Data available

The routine data on need to which we have access are the Korner returns and vital statistics. For non-inpatients, Korner returns provide counts of new contacts in consultant outpatients and with other professional groups separately. This results in double counting, and does not reflect the multidisciplinary teamwork of psychiatric services. As the data is not patient-based, district of residence cannot be identified, though this will change with the new data requirements of the White Paper. In addition to Korner data the Bletchley team have kept a manual register of cases. Also available locally are data on numbers of people on long-acting depot medication, and the numbers of people compulsorily detained under the Mental Health Act. The Health Services Indicators package provides interdistrict comparisons.

A framework for assessing need

Needs assessment can range from the most sophisticated, which is local population based surveys, through to the most crude, but nevertheless useful, which is simply local knowledge of under- or over-provision of services. To develop indicators of need that are of value locally however we need to have access to data that can identify district of residence.

Figure 1 Applying a model
DATA USED

- Korner data
  Non-inpatients
  Inpatients
- Health Services Indicator package
- Mortality statistics
- Demographic characteristics
- Locally collected
  Numbers on depot medication
  Numbers considered at risk

(i) Utilisation data

Figure 2 Applying a model
FILTERS TO CARE

Levels	Filters
1	People in the community
	↓ ← Illness behaviour
2	People attending general practice
	↓ ← Detection of disorder
3	People recognised by GP
	↓ ← Referral to psychiatry
4	People seen by psychiatric service
	↓ ← Admission
5	People admitted

Figure 3 Applying a model
FILTERS TO CARE

Milton Keynes 1989

Level		MK		Bletchley		Expected
		No.	/1000	No.	/1000	/1000
1	Expected no. in community	—	—	—	—	250
2	Expected no. going to GP	—	—	—	—	230
3	Expected no. recog. by GP	—	—	—	—	140
4	No. seen in MH service	771	6	240	6	17
5	No. admitted	297	2	41	1	6

We attempted to apply our local data to Professor Goldberg's model of filters to care. The lowest population level for which we have any data is level 4, the population getting as far as the psychiatric service. The data are simple counts, not related to resident population, and tell us nothing about case mix and severity. Level 5, the hospitalised population, tells us very little about the need for care, as the admission rates reflect the structure and process of the local services. We have no direct data on levels 1, 2 or 3, though this will change in the future as GPs improve their data collection.

These utilisation data could be used as a pointer for needs assessment if compared to that of other districts. Even if there were no problems with the data, the wide differences in service delivery mean these measures are not very useful. Comparisons between districts with similar socioeconomic profiles, or similar service provision, could well be of value. This could be done through the Health Service Indicator package, but was not explored in our annual report. Another measure provided to us by the Bletchley team is referral rates by general practice. This is again level 4 data, and interpretation is difficult with these crude data. It could point to areas of unmet need or inappropriate referral.

Figure 4 Applying a model
VARIATIONS IN GP REFERRALS

Bletchley 1989
Referrals/1000 patients Actual numbers in brackets
3.6 (25)
4.7 (49)
5.0 (55)
5.2 (15)
6.7 (24)
7.6 (36)
8.2 (97)
*9.3 (53)

*Practice in most deprived ward

(ii) Incidence data

We have not used the data on compulsory detainment in the annual report. This is presumably subject to wide variation due to differences in local practice. Parasuicide is another measure which may reflect the burden of mental illness in a population. As only a small proportion are admitted to hospital, routine data is not helpful here, but surveys in Accident and Emergency departments are relatively easy to undertake.

Suicide rates are collectable and are used widely in annual reports. SMRs are available in the Public Health Common Data Set. Because Milton Keynes has been accused of causing 'New Town Blues' and having a high suicide rate we have been monitoring suicide rates in the district. SMRs in Milton Keynes have been high in men and low in women, and interpretation is therefore difficult. However, as suicide is such an extreme indicator it may not be a reliable indicator of the burden of mental illness in the community.

Figure 5 Applying a model
SMRS: SUICIDE 1985–9

	Male	Female
Milton Keynes	114	87
Oxford Region	93	82
England & Wales	100	100

(iii) Prevalence data

The most challenging work of the psychiatric team is the chronically mentally ill living in the community. Community psychiatric nurses across the whole district keep a record of people on long-term depot medication, and this provides a measure of the prevalence of psychotic illness in the district. The Bletchley team also keep a record of those in contact with the mental health services whom they regard as at risk; living precariously in the community. This information is also about to be collected in the rest of Milton Keynes. It will provide a useful measure, but in order to be comparable the criteria for being 'at risk' will need to be defined and agreed.

Figure 6 Applying a model
PEOPLE AT RISK

Milton Keynes and Bletchley 1989

	MKHA		Bletchley	
	No.	/1000	No.	/1000
People on depot medication	94	0.7	26	0.6
People considered 'at risk'	—	—	65	1.0

(iv) Demographic characteristics

Vulnerability factors could be regarded as a proxy measure of need. The ones collected on a population basis through the decennial census are unemployment, low social class, single parent families, families with 3 or more children under 14 at home. In a rapidly growing and changing city such as Milton Keynes the 1981 data is unlikely to be of relevance now.

Summary

(i) Until person based data is collected, routine data will not provide utilisation data by district of residence.

(ii) Routinely available data only give levels 4 and 5 of the 'filters to care' model. Comparisons between districts of similar socioeconomic profiles and/or similar service delivery could be of value in needs assessment.

(iii) The numbers of people on long-acting depot medication, and of people known to the service and considered 'at risk' (criteria to be defined), are relatively easy to collect and could be of value.

(iv) Other proxy measures of mental illness could be used, such as suicide, and social and demographic information.

Contracting for Mental Health: What is Needed?

Dr Dinshaw Master and Ms Claire Perry

Lewisham and North Southwark Health Authority adopted the Clinical Directorate system five years ago.

Figure 1

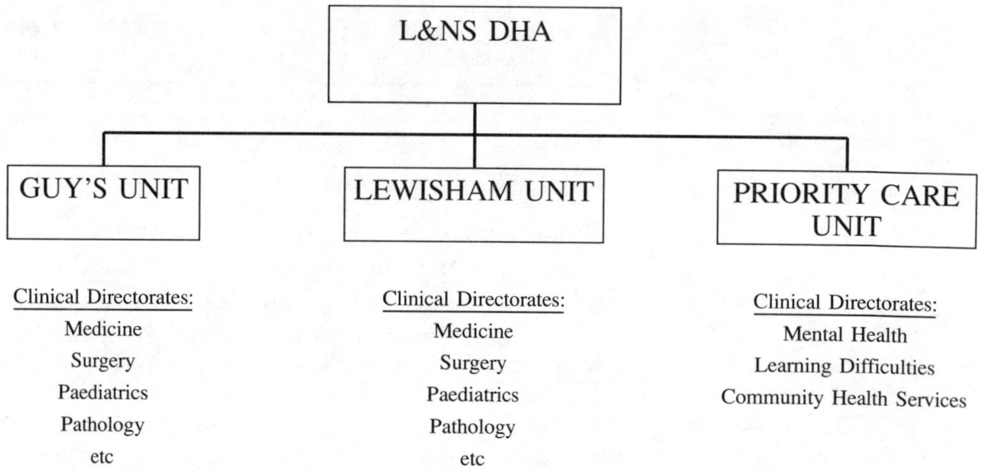

The budget for clinical services is devolved to the three Units of management and Clinical Directorates by the process of negotiating Service Agreements which are in effect contracts between the Directorates and their Units and the District Headquarters. These Service Agreements were developed as simple, realistic annual plans against which service delivery is monitored by Unit and District management boards and by members of the health authority.

Figure 2

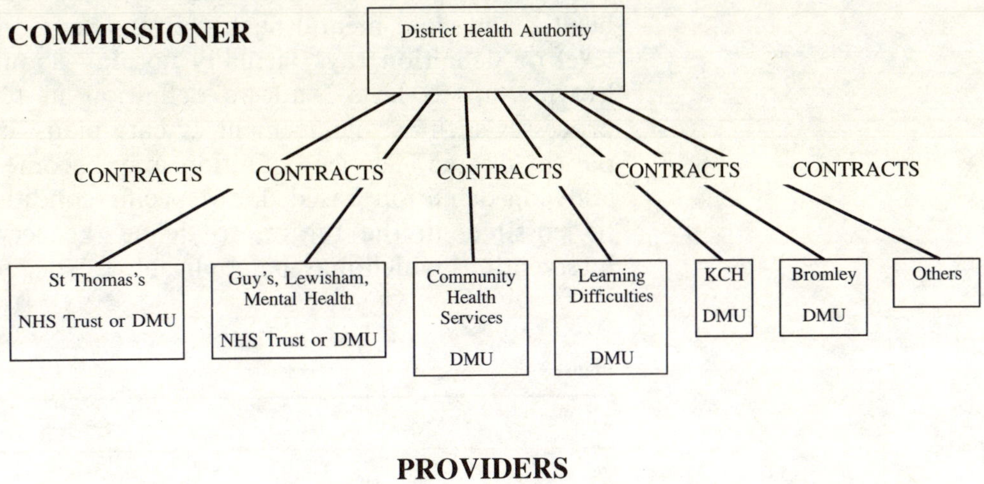

Figure 2 illustrates the future possible contracting scenario for the Lewisham and North Southwark Commissioners. The role of the District Health Authority will change from overall manager of the *services provided* within the boundary to purchasers of services on behalf of *residents* living within the district boundary. The Commissioners will therefore have contracts with their main Provider, the Guy's, Lewisham and Mental Health Services Trust (or DMU) but will also have contracts with other hospital and community Providers for district residents treated outside the district. The Commissioners' role will be to assess the health needs of their residents, to make specifications for the services they will require in order to meet these health needs and to negotiate contracts with a number of Providers.

Figure 3

Service Definition				
1	2	3	4	5
Definition based upon speciality or sub-speciality, eg, AMH, EMH, CMH.		Definition based upon generalised service process (investigation or treatment)		Definition based upon specific investigations or treatment according to condition.

The contract between a Commissioner and a Provider unit contains elements which vary from one clinical service or specialty to another. These are service definition, quality, volume and cost. It also contains elements which are non-variable and which apply across the range of services and specialities. These are the timescale, triggers for renegotiation, methods of payment and monitoring. Service definition, quality, volume and cost may be viewed on a spectrum of sophistication extending from the general to the specific. This is illustrated by portraying these parameters on a scale of 1 to 5. At a primitive level of sophistication (level 1) such as is the case with contracting for mental health services, there is much overlap between these concepts. At an unsophisticated level a service can be described by its component specialities, eg at level 1 mental health services can be defined by their component sub-specialties: adult mental health, elderly mental health, and child mental health. From the Commissioners perspective this level of definition says virtually nothing about what is being purchased. Moving up to level 3 allows definition in terms of generalised service processes such as management or care plans and discharge plans for each patient treated. Service definition may become more sophisticated in time allowing definition based upon specific conditions. Thus at level 5 it may be possible, in the future, to define the service in terms of particular interventions which may be applicable to specific diagnostic groups.

Figure 4

Quality

1	2	3	4	5
Quality defined on basis of structure (eg no. of CPN visits, no. of acute beds, no. of day hospital places)		Quality defined on basis of standards for investigation or treatment (eg ECT procedures adhere to College guidelines; Discharge planning to agreed standard; Referrals seen within agreed time)		Quality defined on desired outcomes (eg ?)

Using the same principle of describing the components of a contract on a spectrum of sophistication, at level 1, quality is defined in terms of structure, which is used as a proxy for quality measures. So the number of CPN visits or the number of hospital beds can be specified in a contract. This not only tells us little about quality, it may also be misleading, eg there may be a great deal of difference between the quality of 12 beds in a back ward of a large hospital and 12 beds in a purpose-built, highly staffed residential unit in the community. Moving onto level 3, quality can be defined in terms of procedural standards, eg ECT procedures which adhere to guidelines issued by the Royal College of Psychiatrists. At level 5, the ideal quality measures would be based on desired outcomes, about which there is much uncertainty in psychiatry. Many may have to do with social outcome, such as the ability to live independently. It may be that the Qalys approach might prove useful but this is at present at an early stage of development (Figure 4).

Figure 5

Volume

1	2	3	4	5
Volume based on historical outputs achieved, eg 800 in-patient episodes, 10,000 out-patient episodes, 75 day patients.		Volume based upon historic activity plus known trends in demand eg residential places increased by 15.		Volume based upon health population profiles and epidemiology

Initially most contracts for mental health services are likely to be block contracts where the Commissioners pay the Provider unit an agreed sum for a defined range of services. For monitoring purposes there would be indicative workloads as illustrated at level 1 (Figure 5). Moving onto level 3, volume could be based on historic activity plus known trends in demand. We are a long way from level 5 where the volume of a contract would be informed by local population profiles and epidemiology.

Figure 6

Cost				
1	2	3	4	5
Lump sum based upon historic activity and costs.		Lump sum based upon packages of care by specialty, volume related.		Per treatment/ investigation cost.

Figure 6 shows this broadly equates with block contracts at level 1, cost and volume contracts at level 3, and cost per case contracts at level 5. Block contracts are likely to be found unsatisfactory because Commissioners will not have details of what they are buying and Providers will be concerned about increasing demand not being matched by increased resources. At level 3 workload agreements are built into contracts. With a cost and volume contract, activity is linked to payment and if the contracted workload is exceeded the contract will specify what additional resources are to be made available probably subject to a negotiated ceiling. At level 5, cost per case contracts are unlikely to be widespread in mental health services, except perhaps for sporadic cases referred from outside the district for specialised treatment.

Figure 7

Contracts will:

- Develop in sophistication over time.
- Develop only at the pace that our information develops.
- Develop at the pace of understanding of health needs assessment and health outcomes.
- Achieve the principles of contracting even if they are not very detailed or specific.
- Need constant attention to be paid to the objectives of contracting.
- Focus on the balance between resources put into a service and the services provided to patients.

Looking at the contracting process using these simple continuums leads to certain conclusions. Contracts will develop in sophistication in time but only at the pace of development of information systems. They will develop only at the pace of our understanding of health needs assessment and outcomes: a particularly underdeveloped area in mental health. Contracts can however be developed at a naive level of information, but we must ensure that our early contracts are based on a clear understanding of how we wish them to develop and that we do not get sidetracked, eg into making our definition of quality structural issues (level 1) more sophisticated, and missing entirely the point of achieving a better understanding of quality outcomes (moving towards level 5) (Figure 7).

Figure 8

Service Provision	*Capability*
• In-patients: 700–800 cases	• Beds: 72
• Out-patients: 9–10,000 attendances	• Revenue: £2,811,000
• Day hospitals: 8–9,000 attendances	• Staff: 155.0 WTE
• Continuing care: 21–24,000 contacts	• Residential places: 15
• Residential care: 15 people	• Bid to DOH for single homeless team revenue
• Day centre: 75 clients	
• Single homeless: 105 clients	

We have found it helpful to lay out our existing service agreements showing the explicit balance required between the services we commit to provide and the use made of the money we receive in return. This allows us to get behind the pounds to examine the use of resources in terms of people, beds, information systems etc to ensure their effective management (Figure 8). The general principle is that nothing should have resources spent on it unless it contributes to services in a specified way. This is a difficult balance to get right but such specificity maximises the chances of achieving this.

Figure 9

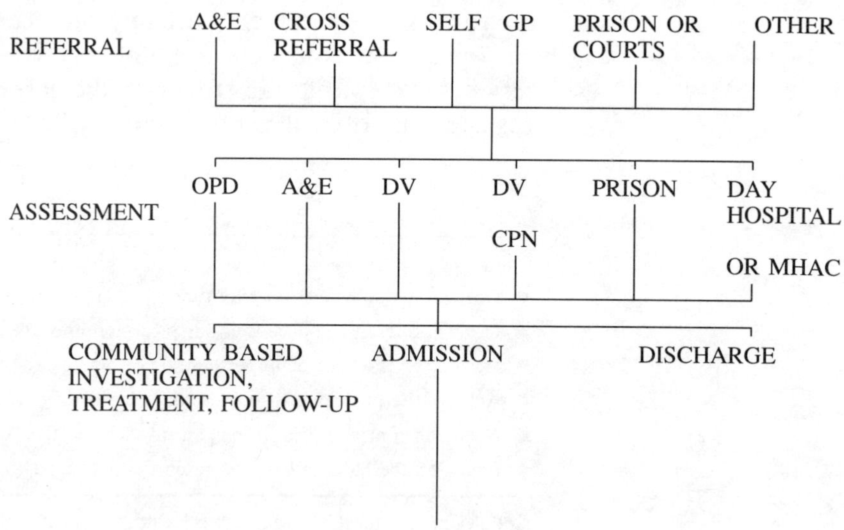

We have used a simple technique of building up a picture of a typical patient through an episode of care. The routes into the service in this example which represents the Adult Mental Health Service are through A&E, cross referral, etc. An assessment follows and the patient is either admitted, discharged or referred to a community-based investigation, treatment and follow-up. Following admission the steps can be mapped out and a full episode of care represented.

Figure 10

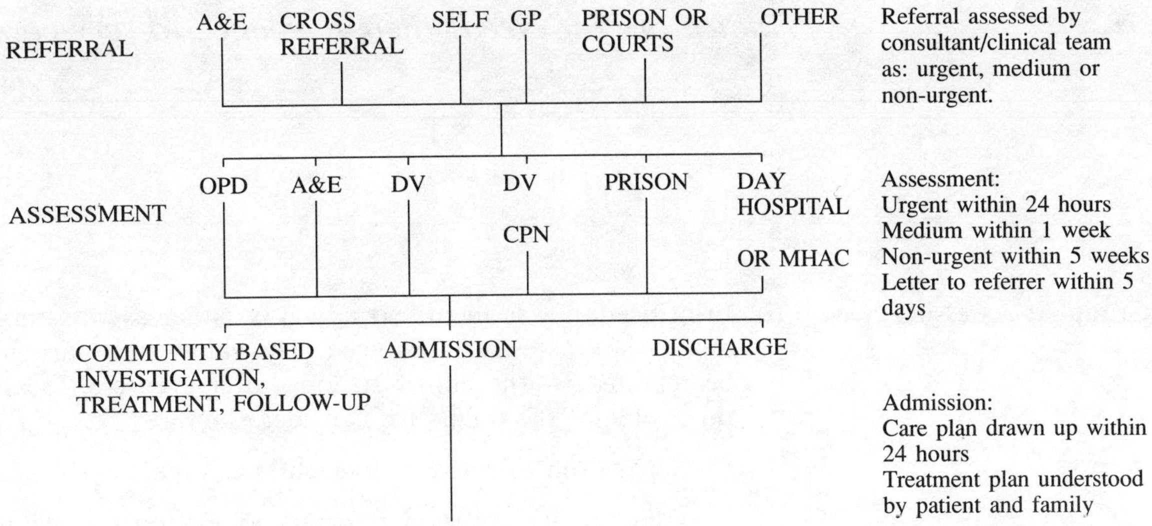

Against each step in the flow diagram the relevant quality standards are committed (Figure 10). This example from last year's service agreement shows some level 1 and 2 structure and process examples. The quality standards will relate to what the Commissioners wish to stipulate and it may be that bodies such as the Royal College of Psychiatrists have a lead role to play in assisting the development and dissemination of such standards.

Figure 11

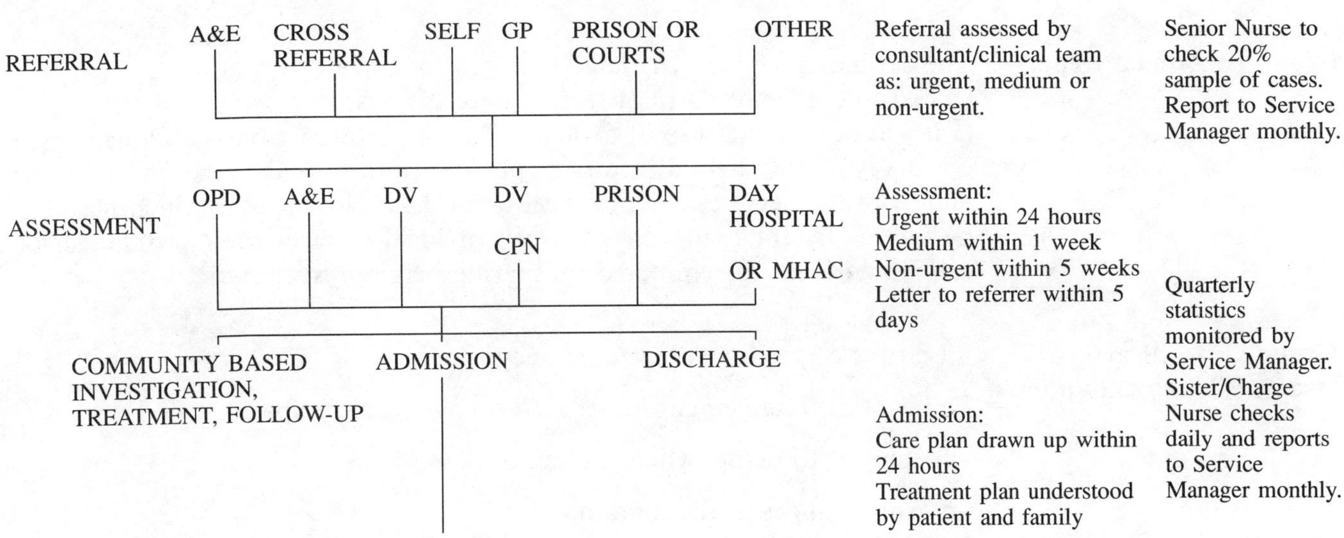

Finally a further column shows the way that Providers will monitor whether the quality standards are being met (Figure 11). Commissioners may have access to this data and may choose to undertake their own monitoring in addition.

In conclusion, this is a view of one way to approach the contracting process. It is an attempt to keep service and quality in the foreground and not to allow contracting to become finance driven.

Discussion from Workshop 1

Indicators for Need: their relevance to service provision

Group A: Assessing Need

(i) Prioritisation was identified as a key issue, as was the need to bring quality into assessment of need. The values of a caring society should be reflected by the ability to look after everyone locally. To achieve this, some of the points for consideration are:

- application of research to each local area
- a comprehensive service for all population groups and between all levels of care
- local decision making
- determination of expected outcomes
- creating a balance between perceived need and demand in planning the service

(ii) Boundaries between primary and secondary care. Needs for:

- GP education and support
- integration of services to allow CPNs and psychologists to work in hospital and community

Group B: Annual Reports

The problems of lack of data, particularly since information systems are geared to the acute hospital sector, were discussed.

It was agreed that use of available data on a district basis complemented by surveys would help directors of public health to make recommendations and prioritise services. Mental health still has a low profile which needs to be raised. By focussing on the work of local services their profile can be raised and ideas disseminated by sharing between districts.

Group C: Contracting Issues. What is a contract?

- a means of getting value for money
- a negotiated agreement ie both sides have to participate
- enables us to define where we are now
- creates changes at the margin

How many contracts?

One for total specialty?

several for different areas?

Some pitfalls in setting contracts:

- no data on quantity
- quality
- cost per case

- purchaser/provider power play

How does the purchaser get advice? From local or outside sources

Quality Structure: Standards are needed for staffing/training

Process: Need to consider ways contracts can ensure dignity, privacy, confidentiality, equality

Outcome: Medical audit is a means of assessing this as is quality assurance. The objective of improved mental health and greater patient independence and satisfaction needs consideration.

Acting measures such as psychotropic prescribing and admission rates are indicators of levels of care but need careful interpretation.

Group D: Indicators of need

- The what and how were discussed including the different approach needed to assess needs for mental health and for mental illness
- standardised advice was required for centrally produced indicators
- indicators could be disaggregated into–
  psychosis
  depression
  dementia
- the white paper agenda focuses on determining need but the public health agenda is wider and focuses on improving the health of the population
- utilization data is a poor proxy for mental health need

Group E: Assessment of unmet need

Areas where surveys would be helpful include prison populations and accident and emergency departments. This will indicate service needs.

- Unmet need does not necessarily mean people are not in contact with services. Some may be in contact with services but receive inappropriate care. Perhaps this group should be a priority for action.

Setting Standards: A Service Blueprint

Professor Eugene Paykel

Abstract

A good psychiatry service needs to provide comprehensive care to a defined population; continuity of care across a range of settings, with fusion of social and medical aspects; a close linking of acute and chronic care; and treatment as near as feasible to the community setting. This is facilitated by a sectorised pattern of service. On the NHS side a considerable range of facilities is required, including inpatient beds, day hospital, outpatient clinics, domiciliary care, and links with primary care. Flexible use is necessary and the possibility of rapid transition between them while preserving a continuity of care. This needs to be supplemented by a wide range of community care facilities for day care (such as day centres, work rehabilitation centres, supportive social clubs), and residential care (including staffed hostels, group homes, cluster flats). Earlier service norms provide useful guides to expected overall provision.

Detailed epidemiological information exists for overall rates of disorder but is usually not available for individual districts. Since psychiatric morbidity tends to parallel social morbidity, the latter provides a reasonable guide to levels of provision required within the range, with modification for the local factors such as differences between different parts of a district, presence of old longstay hospital provision, and problems of accessibility in rural areas.

Needs and Services

Goldberg and Huxley (1980) reviewed pathways and filters on the way to psychiatric care. They estimated that 250 per thousand in the general population might show at least some symptoms of psychiatric disorder. Some would not present to their GPs, others would not be recognised as having psychiatric symptoms, and the majority of the others would receive their treatment by the GP rather than specialised services. From these, about 17 per thousand are referred to the psychiatrist to receive outpatient or inpatient care, and are our main concern today. They are the more severely ill and disabled and are the appropriate targets for specialised services. The apparently alarming numbers of subjects with general practice disorders should not argue for diversion of the current distribution of resources away from the more severe problems handled by the specialised services: most of the general practice patients have mild disorders.

Although psychiatric epidemiology has now provided good information on overall prevalence rates, in practice the epidemiological data do not establish the required psychiatric service provision. This is because most disorder in the community does not require specialist intervention. Measuring prevalence of disorder is not the same as establishing need for treatment.

We finish up using other criteria for deciding on approximate levels and kind of service provision. Epidemiological inferences can then be made to modify provision for one's own district. What this amounts to is starting by looking at what has worked elsewhere, and then if necessary modifying the received wisdom. A useful approach to a local service is to start with provisions elsewhere and national recommendations, to ask how one's own district measures up, and if it deviates, why. There can be very good reasons, but they should be made explicit.

The changes which have taken place so far

The last 35 years have seen dramatic changes in patterns of care, away from the institution and towards the community. There has been a striking drop in occupied psychiatric beds in this country since the mid-1950s from what had previously been a steady rise. This turn-around reflected several factors: new psychotropic drugs, changes in hospital milieus and open doors, rehabilitation, the push towards treatment in the community. Wing (1986) has demonstrated that this drop has particularly been in beds for the old long stay population, occupied for more than 5 years, rather than in short term beds occupied for less than 1 year, or beds occupied for 1–5 years (predominantly for dementia). Outpatient services have shown an equally dramatic opposite trend, with a very marked increase.

Mangen (1985) tabulated numbers of occupied beds per thousand of the population in different European countries in 1979. England and Wales came near the bottom. Different parts of the United Kingdom differed considerably, Scotland having more beds, and Northern Ireland having even more, although some of the difference may reflect the kind of provision for dementia.

Principles of psychiatric service

Principles in the area of service provision are not often made explicit, and this list, although not just my own, is of course selective and far from exhaustive.

Present day psychiatry takes the view that treatment should be based as far as reasonably possible within people's ordinary life and domestic surroundings, rather than in hospital. Psychiatric illness should not disrupt the life of the patient and family any more than can be avoided. To achieve this and an additional aim of accessibility, psychiatric services have to strive as far as possible to be localised. To further this psychiatric services has evolved a pattern of care to a defined geographical locality.

Acute care and chronic longer term care are not easily separable in psychiatry. Many psychiatric patients have illnesses which are recurrent or chronically disabling. Characteristic of most of these long-term disorders is the occurrence of repeated episodes followed by remission and the need for continuity of aftercare following the acute episode to prevent relapse and minimise disability. For many longer term psychotic patients this coexists with impaired awareness of the need for help and inability to press for it, together with particular difficulty in negotiating the stresses resulting from transitions between different settings.

This thus mandates an organisation which permits the team involved with a patient to work flexibly across settings from the hospital to the community, so patients can move easily between these settings without interrupting continuity of care.

Finally, social modes of care are integral to psychiatry and are as important as any other form of treatment. Links with community services are therefore very important to us. Therefore a comprehensive mental health service includes many partnerships between the specialist psychiatric services, and other services factors, general practice, social services, housing authorites, voluntary organisations and self-help groups.

Components of a psychiatric service

The general components and organisation of psychiatric services will be familiar to this audience and are shown in Table 1. The core of a district's psychiatric service is its general adult psychiatry service: what comprises in Department of Health and manpower terms its mental illness service. This

Table 1 Components of a Comprehensive Service

Mental illness (General Adult Psychiatry)
Sectorised general adult psychiatry service
Subspecialities: Rehabilitation
Substance Abuse
(Liaison Psychiatry)
Specialities:
Old age
Mental handicap
Child/adolescent
Forensic
Psychotherapy

will generally nowadays comprise a sectorised service. I will concentrate on its needs in this paper, since I have most practical experience of it.

A particular feature of psychiatric services in this country has been the concept of responsibility for a defined catchment area. Psychiatric hospitals have behaved very differently to general acute hospitals in setting their boundaries in this way. This pattern can look very odd from the outside, but it has considerable advantages. The purpose of a catchment area should not be to forbid the service to people outside it, but to oblige a service to the people who live within it. Psychiatric problems cover a wide range from the congenial young neurotic woman who is said to be a favourite of psychotherapists to the dirty, smelly deteriorated chronic schizophrenic, the unglamorous mental handicapped, and the frightening psychotic murderer. It is very easy for a service to define itself as only serving the more desirable patients, by the process known as upmarketing. Having comprehensive responsibility for a catchment area prevents a service from doing this and obliges it to look after the more disadvantaged patients.

More recently this has been extended to the concept of sectorisation, that is, responsibility for a discrete patch within the wider district catchment area. The very considerable advantages to this pattern are those well known to be associated with localisation of services in general, including ready access, defining of responsibility to a team, and ability to plan what is needed for a defined population. There is also a further advantage. British psychiatry is characterised by the idea of a multi-disciplinary team working flexibly across a range of settings from the hospital to the community to enable patients to move easily between these while retaining continuity and care. This is a triumph of our psychiatric services which we tend not to appreciate. It contrasts markedly with the pattern of separate inpatient, daypatient, outpatient and community facilities operating as independent fiefdoms which is common in many countries, for instance the USA. That pattern makes transitions difficult because there have to be extensive negotiations between autonomous facilities with cumbersome intake procedures. Continuity of care becomes impossible and the concept of responsibility of services to a group of users from the locality fails to operate. Sectorisation produces a different pattern which overcomes these problems.

It is sometimes not popular with general practitioners and it should be used flexibly, the rule being an obligation of responsibility to people from within the sector, but no interdiction to patients from the outside, so that GPs and patients do have some choice. Sometimes choice can be facilitated by twinning teams, or by encouraging each team to develop a special interest.

Officially still part of general adult psychiatry are two subspecialities which require representation at district level: rehabilitation and substance abuse. A modern rehabilitation service will have responsibilities extending across a range of specialised facilities from inpatient units to community residential, day care and work rehabilitation facilities, with a role in planning facilities for longterm care and co-ordinating their operation, including those in the community. This has always been something of a challenge and may be more so in the future.

Substance abuse includes both drugs and alcohol: the facilities may differ, but the modern breed of substance abuse consultants tend to look after both. Alcohol services are now seen as local, and community orientated, rather than Regional.

Liaison psychiatry serving the non-psychiatric parts of the general hospital also needs to be provided, although it does not represent a subspeciality. Some districts, particularly the teaching ones, are moving towards having one psychiatrist with a special responsibility for this service. In other districts, it works well by being shared among all the general psychiatrists, preferably by specific links with individual wards and teams within the general hospital.

Psychiatry has a number of official specialities. Among these, psychiatry of old age has recently emerged as separate from adult mental illness. In earlier planning cycles the two were fused. There are obviously growing needs, and psychogeriatricians are in short supply. The number of Senior Registrar posts has recently been increased, and as they become available, the target is the development of the comprehensive service for the over 65s, except the old longstay chronic schizophrenic population that has crossed the 65 age threshold. The service should span a range of facilities from acute assessment and treatment beds, longer term beds, and community residential and day facilities.

For mental handicap and child psychiatry, services need to be provided in all districts. Modern mental handicap psychiatrists work predominantly in the community, and do not see themselves as responsible for all mental handicap, but only its psychiatric aspects. Some beds will continue to be needed for the mentally handicapped who are psychiatrically ill, or severely disturbed behaviourally.

Forensic psychiatric services need to be available to each district, but have usually been provided so far on a regional basis. Psychotherapy is part of the therapeutic equipment of every psychiatrist. Specialised psychotherapy services have tended to be limited to teaching districts and to concentrate near London, but are increasing.

The Range of Facilities for Adult Mental Illness

Table 2 shows the range of facilities and services which might be expected for adult mental illness within a well-organised district.

I will deal further with levels of provision shortly. A few specific points need to be made about the kinds of provision, starting with the location of acute beds. They should not be too far from the community they serve, if contacts between patients, relatives, and the general community are to be preserved. On the other hand, small distributed units with few beds are very difficult to staff and run effectively. The constraints include medical manpower, since the majority of admissions to acute psychiatric units are emergencies, and these are often after normal working hours. In most districts, the right approach will be to have one, or at the most two, acute admission units for the district.

The advantages of bringing acute psychiatry into the district general hospital are great and have been widely recognised. The move to such units

Table 2 Facilities and Components of a Mental Illness Service

NHS	Other day care	Residential
Inpatient beds	Day centres	Staffed hostels/houses
Day hospital	Sheltered Workshops	Group houses
Community Mental Health centres	Other Work Rehabilitation	Cluster flats
	Social Clubs	
Domiciliary Psychiatrists CPNs	Drop in Centres	
GP		

has been marked and is becoming the general pattern. Sometimes a mental hospital may be situated in the district it serves. Even so, to broaden an isolated service, and to get the greatly reduced stigma and increased quality of care that tend to follow the general hospital location, some of the service will need to be located there. The old Victorian accommodation will in any case need modern replacement and the expense may be incurred on a site that looks increasingly wrong for the future.

Day hospitals are important in psychiatry. A considerable range of acute problems can be treated in them, as well as longer term patients. Controlled studies show that they cannot replace the need for acute admission beds, but they often enable quite short inpatient admission followed by discharge to day care. Day hospitals do need to be near the users, on peripheral sites near the communities which they serve. This may not be easy in rural communities, and the travelling day hospital, which takes its staff to a different local setting, such as a village Church Hall on different days of the week, has been usefully pioneered in West Dorset. This has to be handled carefully since residents of small villages are particularly worried about the loss of anonymity. Even for day hospitals, there needs to be some centrally located provision. Standard recommendations for DGH psychiatric units include a large day hospital, and this seems right. In Cambridge, we have been particularly impressed with the advantages of having the same staff work with the inpatients and the day patients in the same location so that rapid and flexible transition can take place in each direction between inpatient and day patient care, since all that is really different is where the patient sleeps.

Community Mental Health Centres are rather more debatable, and considerably less well defined. A look at those in existence across the country reveals a very wide range of patterns from outreach sites of the main psychiatric service which may even have a few beds, to very autonomous units which may deal with neurotic disorders and interpersonal crises, whose staff particularly value their own independence and keep a pronounced distance from the base psychiatric service. I favour integration, and also careful thought regarding rationale. The best community mental health centre will be the daypatient, outpatient and community care base, situated in a location which is distant from the main psychiatric base so that its residents cannot be well-served otherwise, and operating in close integration with the sector service. The strongest case therefore lies, not in crowded cities, where in fact a large proportion of community mental health centres are situated, but in small rural market towns. Not every district need have a community mental health centre.

Domiciliary work is particularly important for psychiatry and the last twenty years have seen an enormous and welcome expansion in community psychiatric nursing, from a very small start.

Primary care links and services require some discussion. The primary care attachment of community psychiatric nurses has been heavily criticised by Wooff et al (1988) who in Salford found that nurses in primary care did not have a good concept of their roles, were relatively unsupervised, and were carrying increasing caseloads largely of the less disabled. However there is evidence that the psychiatric needs of primary care patients are well met by bringing in outside ancillary workers, such as counsellors, psychologists and nurses. One must be clear that this is really serving the population with minor disorders and is no substitute for adequate care for the more disabled patients requiring specialised services. It is really manpower and resources which impose limitations and oblige a focus on the more disabled.

A recent development has been the growth of work by psychiatrists themselves in primary care. Strathdee and Williams (1984) found that in 1982, one-fifth of all psychiatrists did some work in general practice settings. the figure would be considerably higher today and it has been enthusiastically taken by younger psychiatrists. Some see their outpatients this way; some work with the general practitioner and his team, supervising their work with psychiatric patients. Again the rationale needs to be carefully thought out. It has great value in rural areas, where it is extremely difficult for the patient to travel to the psychiatrist. On the other hand, in cities where there is good public transport and easy access to the outpatient clinic, this may not be the best way to use scarce manpower.

The table also lists a considerable range of community day care and residential facilities, predominantly for the longer term care of the more disabled patients. With the new arrangements for community care, these are the responsibility of the local authority. In psychiatry, we are concerned, since historically psychiatric community care services have come low in the spending priorites of most local authority social service departments, and this is likely to continue in the face of the financial pressures. The gaps have tended to be filled by the NHS, and the creative use of social security funds to support hostels, often fostered by rehabilitation psychiatrists. The arrangements for the mental illness specific grant do give health authorities some role in the future and make the provisions and gaps legitimate targets for Directors of Public Health to include in their reports, where deficits may get some public exposure.

Missing from my list is any mention of prevention. This is a difficult issue in psychiatry. It ought to be very important, but in practice it is not easy to apply at present. The aetiology of mental disorders is not fully worked out; it is often complex and multi-factorial so that primary prevention of a specific disorder by a specific measure may not be possible; it may depend in part on remote childhood experiences. Avoiding these, or even recent stressful events, would require major changes in the way people behave. Primary prevention of functional mental illness is hardly possible at present. Screening might be useful, but it will mainly pick up the milder and possibly self limiting disorders of primary care type, and might simply expand the workload of the service. For mental handicap, by contrast, antenatal screening is of major value, as is genetic counselling. For functional major mental illnesses, secondary prevention, aimed at preventing recurrence and tertiary prevention, aimed at preventing disability, may be more realistic. Crisis centres, helping those reacting to severe life events, may also be helpful. With the exception of mental handicap a major investment in prevention would not be a useful way of spending limited psychiatric resources at present. Pilot projects should have linked evaluative studies.

Amount of service provision

How is one to decide how much to provide of these facilities? It is unfashionable these days to argue from recommended national norms.

However, one does need some externally derived idea of requirements, and previous national recommendations may carry more objectivity than do local enthusiasms.

The most recent national statement recommending levels of provision comes from the DHSS paper "Mental Illness: Policies for Prevention, Treatment, Rehabilitation and Care" (1985). In the 1970s, more the era of national norms, the authoritative recommendations were in the White Paper "Better Services for the Mentally Ill" (1975). The later recommendations only changed these a little. The main outlines are shown in Table 3. Acute bed numbers for under-65s have come down from an earlier recommendation of 50 per 100,000 to a range of 30–50. Psychiatrists have had some reservations about the lower end, depending somewhat on district circumstances and on acceptance that a range implies ability to use the high figure where necessary. Probably the extremes should be extended in either direction in exceptional circumstances. Day places were specified rather confusingly in the 1975 White Paper, which fused together day places for day patients with those occupied by inpatients who might spend their day activities in the DGH unit day hospital space. The total recommendation then was for 65 places per 100,000 of which perhaps 30 might have been used for day patients. The current recommendation is for 40 true day patients per 100,000. It is not entirely clear whether these are envisaged as also including longer term attenders from the community, but day provision is also very important for such chronically disabled patients. Provision for the elderly was set out more clearly in the 1985 paper to include 10 beds per 10,000 over 65 for assessment, which were specified as appropriately located in the general hospital, and about 30 beds for 10,000 for longer stay elderly patients. There is also a recommendation for elderly day places.

Table 3 Recommended Provisions for Adult Mentally Ill and Elderly[1]

NHS (DHSS 1985)	Beds	Day places
Under 65		
Acute	30–50	40
Long Stay	?	?
Elderly		
Assessment/Acute	10	30
Long Stay	30	
Local Authority or other community (DHSS 1975)		
Staffed Hostels	4–6	
Group Homes	15–24	
Day Centres		60

[1] Per 100,000 population (Elderly per 10,000 aged 65+)

Longer term care for under 65s has not so clearly settled into one pattern of service and the plans for it have always been less clear than those for the more acute patients. There is particularly uncertainty as to whether any long stay hospital bed provision is needed for new chronic patients. The various planning documents in the 1970s avoided the issue, although they accepted that some of the old longstay of a previous era were too disabled to be discharged and would remain in hospital until death. It does appear that some severely disabled and disturbed patients are still being generated. The best figures come from the Camberwell Register (Wing 1986) which showed a gradual build up to a stable figure, excluding elderly patients with dementia, of about 50 per 100,000. Although Salford figures are comparable, these are both inner city areas with migration out and the more disabled subjects left behind. Most parts of the country would see fewer such people, down to virtually none in the most favoured areas.

How these places ought to be provided is the unanswered question. In some suitable districts there may be a place for a small unit retained within a mental hospital, but in most areas a better solution would be so-called hospital hostels or hostel wards, ie a house in the community but with 24 hour nursing staffing.

We have lost any explicit recommendations for local authority and other community care provision in the recent recommendations, but I have indicated the figures from the 1975 White Paper. This specified staffed hostel and unstaffed group home places in a range depending on whether the area was one of high or low need. Most of these local authority community places are for longer term care. The 1975 document assumed that this provision would come from the local authority; in the intervening years voluntary and private facilities have come to comprise a substantial proportion on the residential sidc.

Actual Levels of Provision

It is useful to be able to compare oneself not only with recommendations, but with what actually exists in other districts. Up-to-date figures are difficult to come by and the best I can do are figures for 1985, included in the National Audit Office Report on Community Care Developments (1987) which also showed the considerable growth since 1975. These are shown in Table 4. Beds cover under and over 65s, both acute and chronic, including old long stay, so they cannot usefully be compared with the acute recommendations. The NHS day provision of 38 per 100,000 compares with the 1975 recommendation including inpatients of 65. The 16 residential places per 1,000 compares with earlier recommendations of 19–30, which did not explicitly include elderly. The 17 per 100,000 day centre places was far short of the 60 recommended. The community psychiatric nursing provision confirms the spectacular growth of a new specialisation, too small in 1975 for figures to be available.

Further growth should have occurred in all these figures except beds since 1985. If your district far surpasses these provisions it should be congratulated; if it is far short, it should be spurred to act.

Table 4 Provision for Mentally Ill in England 1975 and 1985†

	Places per 100,000	
	1975	1985
NHS Beds	213	161.5
NHS Day Hospital Places	22	38
Residential Places*	8.3	16
LA Day Centre Places	10	17
Community Psychiatric Nurses	2.3 (1981)	4.9

*Local Authority, voluntary and private
†National Audit Office (1987)

Requirements for Staff

With community psychiatric services we move to staffing levels and it is staff rather than facilities which are the most precious assets for a psychiatric service. Here, although the kinds of staff needed are widely agreed, recommendations about levels have been remarkably few. They are most explicit for consultant psychiatrists, partly because the Royal College of Psychiatrists has formulated its own recommendations. The two solid

DHSS recommendations for levels in the 1985 paper were one adult psychiatrist per 40,000 population, and one old-age psychiatrist per district. The College recommendations are not easy to summarise precisely, since some are outdated and some recent, but approximately they are, per 100,000 population: 2.5 adult psychiatrists for a non-teaching district, 4 for a teaching district; 3 sessions of a rehabilitation consultant, some substance abuse time, one each of a child psychiatrist, a mental handicap psychiatrist (formerly 1 per 200,000), and perhaps somewhat idealistically, one forensic psychiatrist and one psychotherapist. The Royal Colleges of Psychiatrists and Physicians jointly recommended in a recent report (1989) one old-age psychiatrist per 20,000 over 65s.

Consultant psychiatrists are only one small component of the staffing of a mental health service and I do not wish to convey any other impression; it is merely that expectations have been formulated. Expected levels for other disciplines have received less specification and are harder for a psychiatrist to come by, although I believe that the Health Advisory Service has some expectations. There was a DHSS target from the 1970s of at least 100 psychiatric nurses per 100,000 population, but this has long been surpassed in most districts. Mangen and Rao (1985) assembled some figures for existing staffing levels in the early 1980s. Per 100,000 population these were 10.3 psychiatrists at all levels (2.6 consultants), 118 psychiatric nurses, 4 community psychiatric nurses, 17 clinical psychologists, 5.4 occupational therapists and assistants. We ought to be doing better now, and we will have to do a lot better still if the wish of the general population for more availability of such staff-intensive treatments such as counselling, psychotherapy, behavioural and cognitive therapies is to be met.

Expectations for the size of a sector in a sectorised service have not been explicitly formulated. My own view is that one team might at present handle 30,000–50,000 total population depending on the setting.

Variations in need

Norms are blunt instruments. They merely suggest an expected average and must be modified in the light of local needs. How should one do this?

The obvious way ought to be from direct knowledge of local epidemiology but this is difficult. Community surveys are too expensive to mount locally and most of the disorder they show is minor. Case registers are difficult and expensive to maintain and they show treated cases which may reflect service provision rather than need. Suicide rates are available, but are of limited value, since absolute numbers are low in any district, and are prone to random fluctuation, as well as not easily explained natural fluctuations. They also need careful interpretation in the light of age and social structure of the population, and local features such as the presence of psychiatric hospitals or hostels catering for high risk populations. Fortunately there are some other easily available indirect guidelines. Some are suggested in Table 5.

Table 5 Some Modifiers of Service Need

Demographic Characteristics
Social Morbidity
Rural Inaccessibility
Local Psychiatric Resettlement

There are obvious demographic correlates of service need, such as the age structure of the population, something well known to South coast planners. Next there is much evidence that major psychiatric morbidity parallels other social and demographic indices, particularly measures of social morbidity. This is particularly the case for schizophrenia which tends to cluster in deprived inner city areas (Bagley et al, 1973). Bed needs in particular are likely to reflect rates of severe psychoses. Not only may rates of disorder be higher, but people in socially deprived areas are also likely to have available fewer alternatives, such as alternative residential provision or private care. Hirsch (1988) suggested that the Jarman indices might provide a useful guide to bed needs, but this really needs validation. The general pattern of looking at social morbidity and thinking in these terms is however a good one. Figures which I published some years ago regarding 1970 psychiatric admission rates nationally by area of residence (Paykel 1978), showed that London had higher rates than the rest of England. Urban inner London had higher rates than suburban outer London; elsewhere, the county boroughs with a more urban make-up had higher rates than administrative counties.

The same lessons apply within a district. The needs of all its parts will not be uniform and most services know pretty well their areas of high and low demand. In Cambridge admission rates for areas within the City of Cambridge, itself fairly genteel by most standards, are about twice as high as those for our rural Fen areas, and outpatient usage also appears to be higher. We are not clear how much this reflects lower morbidity, and how much it reflects higher tolerance of deviance, greater orientation towards psychiatry of city people, or the Fen resident's traditional suspicion of Cambridge, but it does affect the way we need to organise our service.

Rural areas demand further modifications in the delivery of psychiatric services. These have not been as well studied as they ought, and deserve further attention. As already mentioned, day care is not easy to provide. Domiciliary care looms larger, but it is labour intensive and high on travel time and mileage. Appropriate expenditures need to be allowed for.

Another factor modifying needs is presence of a large mental hospital in the district. Although it may provide some margin for beds and an attractive capital land asset for sale, it may also increase the morbidity: there is a considerable tendency which will have operated over many years for discharged patients to settle or be resettled in the area near the hospital they leave.

The factors modifying local needs do also require further study, on a national basis, so that contrasting experiences in different kinds of districts can be more fully analysed.

Annual Public Health Reports

It is not easy to provide indicators for the adequacy of a service and others will deal with this in more detail. Critical evaluation of effectiveness and cost-effectiveness in psychiatric services requires controlled designs, particularly randomised controlled trials, and the use of appropriate outcome measures. These are costly, and it is not feasible to apply them across the board in looking at the standards for a service, rather than at specific questions.

I would suggest that a useful way of starting can be to simply ask the questions: what service provision do we have and how does it measure up? Do we have as much service as other places? Does it show the same pattern or a different pattern? Can we justify the differences rationally and on the basis of local characteristics? What do we lack that we need? Such issues may provide appropriate material for annual reports.

References

Bagley C, Jacobson S and Palmer C (1973) Social structure and the ecological distribution of mental illness, suicide, and deliquency. Psychological Medicine 3, 177–187.

DHSS (1975) Better Services for the Mentally Ill. HMSO.

DHSS (1985) Mental Illness: Policies for Prevention, Treatment, Rehabilitation and Care. HMSO.

Goldberg D and Huxley P (1980) Mental Illness in the Community. The Pathway to Psychiatric Care. Tavistock Publications, London, New York.

Hirsch S R (Chairman) (1988) Psychiatric Beds and Resources. Factors Influencing Bed Use and Service Planning. Report of a Working Party of the Social and Community Psychiatry Section of the Royal College of Psychiatrists. Gaskell Press, London.

Mangen S (1985) Psychiatric policies: developments and constraints. In: Mental Health Care in the European Community, S Mangen (ed.). Croom Helm, London, pp. 1-33.

Mangen S and Rao B (1985) United Kingdom: socialised system–better services? In: Mental Health Care in the European Community, S Mangen (ed.). Croom Helm, London, pp. 228–263.

National Audit Office (1987) Community Care Developments. Report by the Comptroller and Auditor General. HMSO.

Paykel E S (1978) Meeting the needs of mental disorder–in the field of mental illness. Health and Hygiene 1(4), 193–196.

Royal College of Physicians (London) and Royal College of Psychiatrists (London) (1989) Care of Elderly People with Mental Illness. Specialist Services and Training. London.

Strathdee G and Williams P (1984) A survey of psychiatrists in primary care: the silent growth of a new service. Journal of the Royal College of General Practitioners 34, 615–618.

Wing J (1986) The cycle of planning and evaluation. In: The Provision of Mental Health Services in Britain: The Way Ahead, G Wilkinson and H Freeman (eds.). Gaskell, pp. 35–48.

Wooff K and Goldberg D P (1988) Further observations on the practice of community care in Salford. Differences between community psychiatric nurses and mental health social workers. British Journal of Psychiatry 153, 30–37.

Towards a System of Outcome Indicators for Mental Health Care[1]

Dr Rachel Jenkins

Abstract

A system of outcome indicators for mental health care is urgently needed in order to ensure that clinicians, district health authorities, and directors of public health can monitor and evaluate mental health care. Theoretical aspects of health care indicators and the various classes of outcome measures available can be used to draw up a preliminary system of indicators of health care input, process and outcome for the major categories of mental illness, including schizophrenia, affective psychosis, neurosis, dementia, mental handicap, child psychiatry, forensic psychiatry, alcohol and drugs. Such a system is not intended to be definitive or exhaustive but rather to form a basis for development by clinicians, researchers and planners for their own requirements.

The requirement for mental health care outcome indicators

In order to evaluate our health-care system, we need to be able to measure the baseline health of the population, and then to measure the impact of health care on that baseline. We need to be able to monitor and evaluate progress towards more effective health care and better health, to evaluate the efficacy of health-promotion and illness-prevention programmes, and to improve resource allocation in health care. In order to do this effectively in a valid and reproducible manner, health indicators are required. Besides the more global indicators of general health, lifestyles, quality of life, and health equity, we also need indicators relevant to the different categories of illness, and to specific strategies to prevent diseases, to alleviate disability, and to restore function.

While the call for such indicators has hitherto come primarily from planners and policy makers, it should be abundantly clear that indicators are also needed by clinicians if they are in any way to evaluate the effectiveness of their work and to identify areas for improvement, and if district and regional health authorities and organisations such as the Hospital Advisory Service are to monitor quality of service. Particularly urgent requirements at the present time relate to district health authorities (DHAs) and directors of public health. In the 1989 White Paper 'Working for Patients' (para 2: 11), DHAs are asked to:

> 'concentrate on ensuring that the health needs of the population for which they are responsible are met; that there are effective services for the prevention and control of diseases and the promotion of health; that their population has access to a comprehensive range of high quality, value for money services; and on setting targets for and monitoring the performance of those management units for which they continue to have responsibility.'

Thus DHAs in fulfilling their 'purchaser role' will need to develop the ability to monitor service provision, prevention programmes and quality of care, including health outcome.

---

[1] Reproduced with kind permission from ***British Journal of Psychiatry (1990), 157,*** 500–514

There is a danger that measurement will concentrate on those features that are easily quantified rather than those that relate most directly to quality and health outcome. This danger exists in all clinical specialties, and mental health care is no exception. The ability to define and measure quality in mental health services is not well developed. Those aspects of service provision that can most easily be measured at present tend to be those which relate to service input and resources consumed rather than service outcome:

> 'Not surprisingly, most existing mechanisms for external evaluation, such as registration of nursing homes, recognition of training posts, performance indicators, the Health Advisory Service and overseas health service accreditation have focused on resources and process rather than on outcomes.' (Shaw, 1989)

The DHAs will need to construct a population profile that allows health status to be examined over time. In doing this, they will need to draw upon the epidemiological expertise of the directors of public health (see below). Each DHA needs to be able to monitor the quality of services provided by different providers in its area, to measure its progress against other DHAs in the region and nationally, to evaluate new service developments to ensure that objectives are being met, and to encourage each provider to be self-monitoring.

Following the Acheson report (Department of Health, 1988) on the future development of the public health function, the Department of Health issued new guidance to health authorities including the requirement that each district and region should appoint a director of public health (DPH) who must produce each year a report on the health of the population. The DPH is the successor to the medical officer of health, who was removed in the 1974 reorganisation.

The DPH's annual report is an independent assessment of the health of the resident population of the health district or region. The intention is to enable the district or region to discharge its responsibilities in relation to the health of its population. The report should present and interpret epidemiological evidence, identify local health problems including unmet need, and evaluate the outcome of existing services. Its recommendations for action should form an important input to the planning process. The long-term aim should be to reorientate the allocation of resources by health authorities to deal with the identified public health problems.

Indicators as measures

An 'indicator' is defined as a measure that summarises information relevant to a particular phenomenon, or a reasonable proxy for such a measure. Ideally, indicators should actually measure what they are supposed to measure (ie have validity), and they should provide the same answer if measured by different people in similar circumstances (ie have reliability) (Cook & Campbell, 1979). They should be able to measure change (ie have sensitivity), and they should reflect changes only in the situation concerned (ie have specificity) (World Health Organization, 1981). Of course in real life these criteria are hard to achieve, and indicators at best are indirect or partial measures of a complex situation. A *health* indicator, therefore, is a variable, susceptible to direct measurement, that reflects aspects of the state of health of a community, while a *health care* indicator is a variable that reflects aspects of the state of health care in a community (World Health Organization, 1981). Health care indicators can be categorised, using a general systems approach, into input, process, and outcome. The resources put into the health care system in terms of finance, personnel, building, etc., are the input, the activity of the personnel form the process, and the changes in functioning, morbidity and mortality are the outcome. (Thus, in general, outcome indicators in health care will be health indicators.) Outcome may of course be influenced not only by the health care system, but also by other aspects of public policy, social change, and environmental factors.

The measurement of input is relatively straightforward, a simple accounting procedure, and the measurement of process has been tackled for some time, in the shape of 'performance' or 'activity' indicators, although this has sometimes tended to follow the approach of establishing what is collectable first and seeing what it can tell us, rather than specifying the key aspects of performance and devising appropriate indicators.

The measurement of outcome is a more complex task, and the fact that outcome information is hard to obtain has led to health service inputs and processes being used as proxy measures for outcomes, which of course they are not (Bergner *et al*, 1979). It was also argued that because chronic health problems, morbidity and mortality are insensitive variables, and are seemingly unrelated to health care changes in the short term, the use of input and process indicators as proxy measures for outcome was justified. The initial assumption was that use is cure, and amount of use equates with severity of condition, but is now well recognised that use is not necessarily cure, and that utilisation of services varies not only with sociodemographic factors, independent of the severity of symptoms and disability, but also with characteristics of the service, including factors relating to the doctors themselves (see for example Goldberg & Huxley, 1980). This variation greatly compromises the use of services as a proxy for outcome measures of health and leaves us no nearer our goal of measuring the impact of health care on the health of the population.

As we are in an era of relatively easy access to enormous quantities of data, it is vital to give critical thought to how useful the available data are for our purposes of measuring health and monitoring the activities of the health care system (Dean, 1988). It is better first to set priorities, identifying the major health objectives, then to choose the appropriate strategies, and only then to pick indicators to measure the resources that have been applied, how far the strategy has been put into action, and how far it is achieving its objective, than it is simply to use the data that are currently available and let them shape the questions we can answer. It is crucial to understand the meaning of a measure before interpreting it (Bergner *et al*, 1987). For example, one paper commented 'The Goldberg score (derived from the GHQ28) may be considered as an indicator of a premorbid personality disposition towards depression' (Bucher & Gulzwiller, 1988). This is an entirely erroneous conclusion. The GHQ measures the presence of likely depression and anxiety, not personality traits. Indeed, it is specifically designed not to be contaminated by aspects of personality (Goldberg, 1978). Thus, in general, to answer a research question, it is far better to have understood the relationships between the theoretical concepts as far as possible and to use reasonably good indicators, than to use perfect indicators without knowing enough about their relationships (Mootz, 1988). Research must determine the way health is measured, not the availability of complex health indices. Otherwise, exclusive concentration on measurement will limit the conceptual development of the topic, and may inhibit thinking and planning.

Present outcome indicators in health care

The present health indicators that have been used as outcome measures include those of mortality, morbidity (as measured by disability days, bed days or restricted activity days, hospital admission figures), subjective health indicators, direct measures of health and social functioning, and measures of unmet need.

Mortality

This, the most frequently used measure, does not indicate health at all, but lack of survival (Dean, 1988). As a general principle, mortality is an important indicator of social conditions such as road safety and violence, as well as of the treatment of life-threatening diseases, but mortality data do not adequately reflect changes in health status within populations (Patrick & Erickson, 1987). Decreased mortality may not signal a healthier population; on the contrary, it may reflect the longer life of chronically ill and seriously disabled people (Wilson, 1981). In mental illness, there is of course an avoidable mortality, that caused by suicide. The official suicide rate, although known to be an underestimate, is a reasonable indicator of all deaths from suicide (Sainsbury, 1983), but it is not a good indicator at all of rates of mental illness. However, overall mortality rates, not just those of suicide, may be a helpful indicator of the adequacy of health care for mentally ill people. Fox & Goldblatt (1982) have demonstrated the grossly elevated standard mortality rates (SMRs) of people in the years following their discharge from mental hospital, largely due to cardiovascular and respiratory disease, presumably reflecting poor social and medical care.

Morbidity

Disability days, bed days, and restricted activity are indicators which may reflect many conditions other than health, such as provision for paid sick leave, the number and age of children in a family, and the division of responsibilities within families, as well as psychosocial factors such as the tendency to assume a sick role or to express problems through somatic symptoms. Disability days are more properly regarded as a measure of social disability (Wilson, 1981). However, they are useful, for example, as a measure of self-care during illness. (It is worth remembering that in a prospective investigation of 6,928 adults, a pattern of greater mortality was found among persons with no disability days in comparison with those who reported one to three sick days during a year (Berkman, 1975); the greater mortality of people with no sick days was independent of age, sex, objective and subjective health status, and health habits.)

Bed usage and hospital admission/discharge figures are not in themselves outcome indicators because they are affected not only by the availability of beds, but also by:

(a) inflow factors, such as the availability of alternative services (eg day hospitals or community psychiatric nurses could reduce the need for admission)
(b) factors influencing length of treatment, such as the admission of heavily dependent patients when alternative arrangements in the community take a long time to set up, or the special interests of the team (eg a brief admission policy, the admission of forensic cases under a court order, in-patient psychotherapy)
(c) outflow factors, which influence the transfer of patients back to the community or to other appropriate units.

If these factors are explored and understood, then admission figures can become helpful to us in monitoring interventions to rationalise inflow, length of stay, and outflow. However, psychiatric in-patients represent only 1–2% of the total of psychiatric morbidity. In mental illness, as with other medical conditions of varying severity such as asthma or hypertension, not all cases reach hospital or even come to medical attention. It is therefore important for us to develop health indicators that apply not only to hospital in-patients, but also to the rest of the iceberg of morbidity in the community. Similarly, we need input and activity indicators not only for hospital services, but also for the primary-care services.

Subjective health indicators

These are measures that focus on experiential aspects of illness, distress and discomfort, instead of the more objective evaluation of health status by a professional. They are important to consider because of the research evidence that self-perceived health correlates with mortality and rate of recovery even after controlling for objective measures of health. Furthermore, subjective measures of health correlate more closely with use of health services than do the medical conditions themselves (Hunt, 1988). There is often a disparity between judgements of professionals and lay people on whether a particular treatment has been successful, and it is crucial to take the lay view as well as the medical view.

Direct measure of health and social functioning

These have by far the strongest conceptual basis as relevant indicators of health outcome. Many measures have separate physical, psychological, and social axes, while there are also combined measures, including measures of quality of life. It is not appropriate to describe these measures in detail here, but good reviews are available (eg McDowell & Newell, 1987; Thompson, 1989). Some measures assess positive health as opposed to ill health, presumably pursuing the World Health Organization's (1948) definition of health as 'a state of complete physical, mental and social well being and not merely the absence of disease or infirmity'. While the fact is that the National Health Service's overwhelming present task is to wrestle with the cure and prevention of illness and handicap, and with the delivery of care to the sick, and this should be its first objective, the pursuit of 'positive' health is not just a fanciful notion.

The importance of positive health is that it is typically used to describe some aspect of lifestyle or mental outlook that is associated with better future health. For example, a person with refined skills for coping with stress may not differ from others without such skills at the present time, but this person may have a higher probability of better mental and physical functioning in the future. However, it would be entirely premature to move from indicators of 'negative health' to those of 'positive health' (Bice, 1979).

Unmet need

'Unmet needs' have been defined as the differences between those services judged necessary to deal appropriately with defined health problems and those services actually being received. Changes in unmet need are measures of the outcome of health services, but they are not in themselves measures of health status (Carr & Wolfe, 1979). They do not measure the level of health of an individual or a population but rather they measure the capacity of the health and social care system to care for the sick. There is a strong tradition of measuring unmet need in the US, reviewed by Carr & Wolfe (1979), which has been developed by Brewin *et al* (1987, 1988) for mental illness. Indicators for unmet needs and health care outcome, although not the same, are related. Indicators for unmet needs relate to the services and resources necessary to maintain and improve health status. Carr & Wolfe

(1979) suggested that the provision of appropriate health services according to need is an intermediate outcome of a health system whose ultimate goal may be to improve the health status of a population.

Global indicators

Some investigators have attempted to define a single 'gross national product' of health status, by combing data on mortality, morbidity, disability, and even health expenditure in various weighted ways into a health status index. Unfortunately such an approach tends to obscure rather than inform, because information about health must serve different purposes. In order to answer specific questions, the index has to be disaggregated into its component parts. It has been claimed that the loss of detail accompanying aggregation is offset by the increased generality of application. However, Bice (1979) argues that the history of measurement supports the view that progress is marked by increasing ability to discriminate between quantities and qualities of phenomena, and not by devising qualitative summaries that obscure differences.

Social indicators

The social dimension of health and the health care system must not be ignored, and Gulbinat (1983) pointed out that, in addition to direct measures of mental health, we need indicators of psychosocial development from childhood to old age, and also of social pathology (including family disruption and lack of social support). Some indicators of social pathology are readily available, such as the crime statistics and rates of divorce, illegitimacy, homelessness and unemployment, although there are the usual problems of interpretation, under-reporting, and changing cultural life-styles, which negate the value of some official statistics (for example many couples may successfully cohabit for a number of years without entering the marriage statistics). Indicators of psychosocial development pose a much more difficult problem, but they should at least take into account age-specific and stage-specific problems, which have their own measurement requirements (Siegmann, 1979).

Demographic indicators

Finally, since health policy does not only aim to improve the average level of health but also to reduce inequalities in health among the various subgroups of a population, we not only need indicators of the level of health of the general population, but also an assessment of the differentials among population subgroups. This means that we also need a coherent strategy for applying health indicators across the nation, so that there is agreement on the subgroup definitions, which may be socioeconomic, ethnic, geographical, etc.

The need for research

While indicators can tell us about the quantity of mortality or morbidity, and can measure change over time, it is important to be clear that they cannot in themselves attribute change to a specific cause—it would be necessary to carry out carefully designed research projects which control for the other extraneous variables. Therefore it is vital to develop and test health indicators in the context of appropriate research projects to monitor health and health-promotion programmes (Culyer, 1983; Hansluwka, 1985; Lohr & Ware, 1987). Furthermore, there is a need for a closer dialogue between researchers and policy makers, leading to the notion of integrated health policy and research, in which responsibility is shared equally between the researcher and the end-user (Noack & McQueen, 1988).

A preliminary consideration of outcome indicators

This paper presents a brief consideration of indicators of health care input, process and outcome of schizophrenia, affective psychosis, neurosis, dementia, child psychiatry, forensic psychiatry, mental handicap, alcohol and drugs; it is not intended to be definitive or exhaustive but rather to form a basis for development by clinicians, researchers and planners for their own requirements.

Schizophrenia

Districts confront a life-time risk of schizophrenia of approximately 1% in the adult population, and while a third of cases do well, the remainder have repeated relapses and readmissions, and at least half of these undergo severe deterioration.

Before setting objectives, it is helpful to ask some preliminary basic questions.

Can the incidence of schizophrenia be reduced?

The aetiology of schizophrenia may be at least half genetic (Rosenthal, 1971), probably due to a polygenic rather than a single-gene mechanism (Cutting, 1985). Rainer (1982) quotes the life-time risk of developing the disorder as 10–15% for a child with one schizophrenic parent. Therefore adequate access to simple genetic counselling (by ensuring the education of primary-care and secondary-care teams to provide this on request) and the availability of contraceptive services may help a little in the long term (Reveley, 1985).

Can relapse rates and readmission rates be reduced?

Research has demonstrated that the delivery of family interventions (which reduce those family stresses and conflicts that precipitate relapse and readmission) and direct education of sufferers about the management of their own illness, can dramatically reduce relapse rates and readmission rates (Falloon *et al*, 1982, 1985; Leff *et al*, 1985; Birchwood *et al*, 1989).

Can total disability be reduced

Research has demonstrated that the provision of adequate rehabilitative services can have a major impact on total disability (Wing, 1982), and that the accretion of severely dependent patients is much lower in the presence of such services (Hyde *et al*, 1987).

Is there an avoidable mortality?

Ten per cent of schizophrenics commit suicide (Hawton, 1987) and their SMRs are grossly elevated from those in general medical illness, including cardiovascular and respiratory diseases (Fox & Goldblatt, 1982), presumably contributed to by smoking, poor nutrition, poor environmental conditions, and lack of adequate medical and social care.

Objectives

These would therefore include:

(a) to reduce the incidence of schizophrenia
(b) to reduce relapse rates and readmission rates
(c) to reduce the total disability and deterioration in social functioning
(d) to prevent patients from 'falling through the care net'
(e) to reduce the suicide rate
(f) to reduce the premature mortality from all causes, especially cardio-vascular and respiratory disease
(g) To reduce unemployment
(h) to provide satisfactory housing
(i) to continue research into the causes, consequences and care of schizophrenia.

Input indicators

These would be:

(a) genetic counselling services within the framework of both primary and secondary care
(b) social support for vulnerable people and families
(c) family interventions
(d) direct education of sufferers
(e) adequate rehabilitation services, including housing where necessary, and case-management systems
(f) education of primary-care and secondary-care teams about suicide risk
(g) adequate primary physical health monitoring
(h) adequate employment opportunities
(i) care registers to facilitate action and communication by secondary-care and primary-care teams.
(j) active research on the causes, consequences and care of schizophrenia.

Process indicators

Indicators of activity on all the above factors would be required.

Outcome indicators

These would include:

(a) prevalence figures from the local psychiatric services register, together with grading of levels of disability, and supplemented by local-community research surveys
(b) hospital first-admission and readmission rates
(c) employment rates in local schizophrenic patients
(d) prevalence of suicide in local patients
(e) SMRs of patients with schizophrenia
(f) prevalence of homeless in local schizophrenic patients.

Affective psychosis

The life-time risk of affective psychosis is approximately 1% of the adult population; the illness is severe and recurrent, but it does not generally lead to deterioration between episodes. It can be treated and relapses can be minimised by the use of prophylactic drug therapy.

Again, before setting our objectives, it is helpful to ask some preliminary questions.

Can the incidence of affective psychosis be reduced?

The aetiology of affective psychosis is at least partially genetic (Reich *et al*, 1982). Morbid risk in relatives varies with unipolar and bipolar illness, age of onset, and responsiveness to treatment.

Can relapse rates and readmission rates be reduced?

These can be reduced by prophylactic drug therapy, and by adequate early-warning communication between family, primary-care and secondary-care teams and by the provision of adequate social support (Bennett, 1982).

Can total disability be reduced?

The disability is generally far less than for schizophrenia, as deterioration of personality does not occur in the same way, and multiple handicaps are less likely to accumulate. Adequate occupational opportunities are crucial after recovery (Bennett, 1982).

Is there an avoidable mortality?

Fifteen per cent commit suicide (Miles, 1977). Continuing education of primary-care and secondary-care teams in how to assess suicidal risk is vital if the rates are to be reduced.

Objectives

These would therefore include:

(a) to reduce the incidence of affective psychosis
(b) to reduce relapse rates and readmission rates
(c) to reduce the suicide rate
(d) to reduce the premature mortality from all causes
(e) to maximise employment
(f) to eradicate homelessness
(g) to continue research into the causes, consequences and management of affective psychosis.

Input indicators

These would be:

(a) genetic counselling services within the framework of primary and secondary care
(b) continuing education of primary-care team about risk and advantages of prophylactic drug therapy
(c) continuing education of primary-care and secondary-care teams about assessment of suicide
(d) adequate primary and physical health monitoring
(e) adequate employment opportunities
(f) care registers to facilitate action and communication by care teams
(g) active research into the causes, consequences and management of affective psychosis.

Process indicators

These would be indicators of activity on all the above factors.

Outcome indicators

These would include:

(a) prevalence figures from the local psychiatric services register, supplemented by local community research services
(b) hospital first-admission and readmission rates
(c) employment rates
(d) prevalence of suicide in local patients.

Neurosis

Districts confront depression and anxiety as very common disorders, occurring in about 10–25% of the adult population (depending on the threshold adopted for 'caseness'). Half recover in a few months, the remainder pursue a variable chronic course which may last two years or more. Although these conditions are not psychotic, and although some are minor, others are severe and handicapping, with damaging consequences for the sufferer and the wider community. Most should be readily treatable in primary care. Depression is used as an example.

Can the incidence of depression be reduced?

The causes of non-psychotic depression are environmental rather than genetic (Torgensen, 1983; Jenkins, 1985). Some depression is secondary to physical disease, pain and disability, and is helped by the prevention and treatment of physical disease, pain and disability (particularly loss of mobility and sensory function) (eg Cooper, 1976). Some cases of depression are precipitated by acute life events and can be prevented by crisis intervention, and other systems of support (Newton, 1988). Some is precipitated by lack of social support and can be prevented by setting up systems for at-risk groups (eg isolated mothers of pre-school children). Organisations such as CRUSE and NEWPIN, as well as adequate child and family psychiatric services, may all help.

Can recovery rate be improved?

The prognosis can be improved by improving the detection and treatment of depression in general practice. Research has shown that depression detected by the general practitioner (GP) has a better prognosis than 'hidden' morbidity (Johnstone & Goldberg, 1976). At present GPs only identify about half of the total morbidity (Goldberg & Huxley, 1980).

Is there an avoidable mortality?

A small proportion of depressed people commit suicide, and the risk of death from all causes including accidents is twice the norm in severe neurotic depression (Sims & Prior, 1978)

Objectives

These would therefore include:

(a) to reduce the incidence of depression
(b) to increase detection rates by primary-care teams
(c) to reduce chronicity of depression
(d) to reduce the premature mortality from all causes
(e) to continue research into the causes, consequences and care of depression, particularly in primary care.

Input indicators

These would be:

(a) adequate screening and treatment facilities in primary care for physical disease and disability, loss of morbidity and sensory function

(b) system for primary-care teams to identify those in their practice populations who are particularly at risk, including the elderly, young, isolated mothers of pre-school children, the disabled, and informal carers of severely physically ill or mentally ill patients, and to screen regularly, either opportunistically, or on home visits where appropriate

(c) resource indexes in primary care, listing sources of support for their practice population

(d) counsellors, psychologists and social workers in primary health care

(e) 'stress' programmes in local workplaces, with good collaboration between industry and health care teams

(f) adequate training in detection (and treatment where appropriate) of depression for primary-care teams, social services, and occupational health services

(g) active research studies on the causes, consequences and care of depression, particularly in primary care.

Process Indicators

These would be indicators of activity on all the above factors.

Outcome indicators

These would be:

(a) community surveys

(b) general practice identification index

(c) prevalance of suicide and parasuicide.

Dementia

Dementia involves an irreversible decline in cognitive faculties, ending in death. It occurs in 20% of those aged over 80.

Can incidence be reduced?

The incidence of arteriosclerotic dementia can be reduced by factors reducing arteriosclerosis. The incidence of senile dementia cannot at present be reduced.

Can functioning be improved?

Functioning of demented people can be improved significantly by various general measures: appropriate support for living in the community, to prevent admission to institutions with its attendant risks of decompensation of dementia, depression, decreased mobility, and death; and adequate training and support for carers in the community and in institutions, particularly in the recognition of depression and toxic confusional states.

Is there an avoidable mortality?

Life expectancy is five years for senile dementia, and two years for arteriosclerotic dementia, and at present little can be done to improve mortality rates.

Objectives

These would include:

(a) to maximise functioning
(b) to reduce the incidence of depression and toxic confusional states
(c) to ensure adequate training and support to all carers, both formal and informal
(d) to continue research into the causes, consequences and care of senile dementia.

Input indicators

These would include:

(a) adequate support services (eg home-helps, laundry services, incontinence services, meals, medical checks, attendance at day centres, lunch clubs, adequate chiropody, physiotherapy, and mobility, aids for deafness and blindness)
(b) night nursing and respite care, to support informal carers in their task
(c) adequate training and support for informal and formal carers, particularly in recognising treatable conditions such as depression and toxic confusional states which will otherwise greatly reduce functioning
(d) availability of a range of institutional care when necessary (eg Part-III accommodation, nursing homes, day care)
(e) active research in the causes, consequences and care of senile dementia

Process indicators

These would include indicators of activity on all of the above.

Outcome indicators

These would include:

(a) community and institutional surveys of prevalence and severity of dementia, depression and toxic confusional states
(b) admissions to institutional care and day care.

Child psychiatry

The two major disorders of childhood are emotional disorders and conduct disorders (occurring in one in ten children and one in five adolescents) (Rutter, 1989). Psychosis in childhood is very rare (less than 1 per 1,000).

External influences are as important as the child's temperament and character. Clearly, individuals differ in their resilience to environmental stresses. Different undesirable experiences may have different risk potentials for cognitive, socio-emotional and behavioural development (Kolvin *et al*, 1990). In the last two decades the developmental process has been seen as more fluid than before, and dependent on the interaction of genetic and environmental processes at all stages, from the intrauterine environment to the psychosocial environment of the school. There has been a considerable growth in research into both the genetic and environmental transmission of child psychiatric disorder (Earls & Jung, 1987)

Can incidence be reduced?

Sociocultural factors play an important role in the incidence of emotional and conduct disorders, and it is likely the greater our understanding of the way such factors influence emotion and behaviour, the easier it will be to reduce their incidence.

Mentally handicapped children have a higher rate of psychiatric disorder, possibly three to four times higher than that found in a randomly selected control group (Rutter *et al*, 1970*a, b*). Factors lowering the incidence of mental handicap will lower the incidence of psychiatric disorder overall.

The child psychiatric disorders that follow head injury can be reduced in incidence by improved prevention of head injury, for example by wearing an adequate helmet when cycling, better car seat-belt legislation, etc. We know some of the specific risk factors with regard to psychiatric disorder in childhood and adolescence, such as organic brain dysfunction, lead toxicity, and family discord. We know that the school and the area of residence both have influences on the onset of psychiatric disorder.

Other evidence suggests that environmental deprivation can be prevented by a network of social and emotional supports, especially in the pre-school years, ensuring good maternal health, an absence of financial and employment problems, encouraging a small family size, and helping women to wait until they are emotionally mature before becoming mothers.

Can relapse and readmission rates be reduced?

Very few children in fact require hospital admission. Rates are subject to the same factors as in general adult psychiatry. However, disturbed children and adolescents may be admitted to educational or social services facilities as well as hospitals.

Can total disability be reduced?

There is evidence that total disability can be reduced, but not to what extent.

Is there an avoidable mortality?

The two psychiatric conditions most associated with death in this age group are suicide and overt anorexia nervosa, although both are rare. Death from child abuse is related to parental psychopathology, but abused children may be referred to a child and adolescent psychiatry service (those deaths are usually prevented by vigorous interventions by health, social services and the court).

Major depression and suicide constitute an increasing public health problem among the young. Risk factors for suicide are: male sex, depression, intoxication, previous suicide attempts, and ready access to the means. Early detection and amelioration of depression, appropriate and early intervention for parasuicide, and controlling the commonly used methods of suicide (eg drugs and guns) are likely to reduce the suicide rate.

Objectives

These would include:

- (a) to reduce the incidence of psychiatric disturbance
- (b) to reduce rates of relapse, where applicable
- (c) to reduce the rates of hospital readmission
- (d) to reduce the parasuicide rate
- (e) to reduce the suicide rate
- (f) to reduce educational failure due to psychiatric disturbance
- (g) to improve the quality of life for those children caught in psychosocially disadvantaged families

(h) to reduce the impact of social deprivation and emotional deprivation
(i) to improve the detection of those likely to develop chronic illness
(j) to continue research in this specialty.

Input indicators

These would include:

(a) improved training of medical undergraduates and GP postgraduate training to enhance the ability of GPs to detect psychiatric disturbance in children and adolescents and to know when to refer those to specialist services
(b) provision by health visitors of a service to families with pre-school-aged children, as by nursery nurses, play-group leaders
(c) provision by teachers, school welfare officers and education psychologists of a service to school children (and some identified pre-school children), and by the school health services employees
(d) provision by social workers of counselling services to families, and their statutory duties to provide care and protection for some children at risk
(e) specialist services offered by child and adolescent psychiatrists, child psychotherapists, clinical and educational psychologists, and other therapists, eg speech therapists, physiotherapists, drama therapists
(f) specialist health facilities, including out-patient, day-patient and in-patient services, on a district, regional or supraregional basis, according to need as well as financial and manpower resources (of special note are the two youth treatment centres–the adolescent forensic service provided by the Gardner Unit at Prestwich Hospital, and the Young Persons Unit in Ashworth Hospital)
(g) additional specialist educational services, such as special day and residential schools
(h) additional specialist social services, such as community homes (with or without education provided on the premises), assessment centres, the Aycliffe Institute for Adolescent Disorders
(i) independent organisations providing counselling and psychotherapy services, in-patient and out-patient services and residential homes
(j) extensive research conducted nationally and internationality.

Process indicators

These include indicators on activity on all the above factors.

Outcome indicators

Outcome, in this field, is not always measureable clinically; for example a request to write a report for the court will have a legal outcome. Often the outcome is a *social* one and not a health one. Change can be seen as 'dynamic' change or 'symptom' change. Some indicators are:

(a) measures of function (a dynamic change, eg learning better)
(b) symptoms reduced in severity or frequency
(c) symptoms removed
(d) prevalence rate reduced
(e) rate of attempted suicide reduced
(f) rate of completed suicide reduced
(g) chronic disturbance detected at an early stage
(h) readmission rate for serious disorders reduced
(i) rate of reception into care reduced (a social outcome)
(j) delinquency prevented or the rate of police involvement/court appearances reduced.

Forensic psychiatry

District health authorities have a responsibility for the care of mentally disordered offenders who originate from their district. The prevalence of mentally disordered offenders in the general population is unknown, although the prevalence in prison populations has been variously described as between 4% and 20%. Of the resident population in all mental illness and mental handicap hospitals on 31 December 1986, 2.5% were detained under the criminal provisions of the Mental Health Act 1983 (unpublished Home Office calculation). A relatively small group of psychiatric patients have many problems: unemployment, homelessness, often intractable and severe mental disorder which has left social handicaps, behavioural problems, and potential for reoffending. As with all ex-psychiatric patients, the SMRs are elevated. This group often requires management by a combination of psychiatric teams, probation services, prison services, prison medical service, social work, general medical and general practitioner teams, as well as appropriate liaison with police, courts, Crown Prosecution Service and solicitors acting on behalf of their clients.

Can the numbers of mentally disordered offenders be reduced?

Mental illness (above) and mental handicap (below) are discussed in other sections, so this section concentrates on personality disorder (the commonest psychiatric condition associated with persistent offending), where it is possible that incidence could be reduced. Illegal delinquent acts are common (80% of all boys). Only a minority become persistent adult offenders. A number of environmental factors significantly increase the chance of becoming persistently delinquent: bad parenting, criminal fathers, alcoholic parents, low IQ, low family income, and large family (West & Farrington, 1977), and school (Rutter & Giller, 1983). Early identification of vulnerable people and families with appropriate interventions by caring agencies (training for parenthood, medical help for alcohol problems, social services and probation services support, school awareness, etc.) may help to reduce the incidence. Rutter & Giller (1983) showed that a number of factors may protect a person against delinquency: a good peer group (eg at school), successful employment, a good marriage, an improvement in life circumstances, one good relationship, good life experience outside the home (eg at school).

Can relapse rates and readmission rates be reduced?

For personality disorders, counselling and general support (probation and out-patient services) seem to help, although this is stated on the basis of clinical experience rather than research. It certainly seems to assist in preventing reoffending, in some people. Patients may well develop insights into their difficulties, which will help them successfully manage stressful events in their lives.

For mentally disordered offenders, careful follow-up after discharge from a regional secure unit has been shown to result in less time spent in hospital and less reoffending during the two years after admission compared with the two before (unpublished DHSS study).

Can total disability be reduced?

There is a tendency for maturation to take place with time. This is probably helped in some cases by general support and counselling, which lead to greater ability on the part of the patient to cope. Treatment in special therapeutic communities (eg Grendon Prison) is thought to help, especially with younger, more intelligent psychopaths–but again, there is not a controlled trial to establish this. Research suggests that on return to the original environment, the benefits of the more structured setting are lost (Gunn *et al*, 1978).

Is there an avoidable mortality?

About 5% of people with psychopathic disorder commit suicide. Those with personality disorder are often said to be more reckless and to have a higher death rate from accidents.

Objectives

These would include all the objectives given under 'Schizophrenia' and 'Mental handicap'. Additional objectives would include:

(a) reduce the incidence of mentally disordered offenders
(b) reduce the incidence of personality disorder
(c) reduce reoffending rates, as well as relapse and readmission rates
(d) reduce suicide rates
(e) reduce premature mortality
(f) prevent entry and re-entry into criminal justice system
(g) reduce the social handicaps
(h) reduce unemployment
(i) reduce homelessness.

Input indicators

These would include, as well as those for schizophrenia and mental handicap:

(a) systems to identify vulnerable people and families, and deliver social support, health services, probation services, school support, and pre-parenthood training
(b) systems to provide psychiatric services for assessment, and advice to courts, police stations, Crown Prosecution Service, probation services, and to provide early diversion from the criminal justice system
(c) systems to provide psychiatric service to prisons, to aid transfer of mentally disordered prisoners to hospital
(d) systems to ensure ongoing support and care from psychiatric and other services on release from prison
(e) systems to ensure rehabilitation, and to facilitate multi-agency management (eg assessment panels)
(f) access to housing
(g) adequate employment opportunities.

Process indicators

These would be indicators of activity on all above factors.

Outcome indicators

These would include:

(a) numbers of patients detained under Section IV of the Mental Health Act 1983, and their admission and readmission rates.
(b) prevalence of treatable mentally disordered offenders in prison population
(c) numbers of patients diverted from criminal justice system (not collected at present)

(d) suicide rate in prison (overall rate in 1987 was 39 per 50,265 prisoners)
(e) SMRs.

Mental handicap

The prevalence of mental handicap varies according to the degree of handicap and to age, but an overall prevalence of severe mental handicap is 3–4 per 1,000. Mild mental handicap is found in 20–30 per 1,000. The incidence of severe mental handicap is 5.4 per 1,000 live births. It is thought that 1.5 per 1,000 people with mental handicap are at risk of developing a mental illness (Corbett, 1979). Day (1983) suggested 0.25 beds per 1,000 people were required for a comprehensive psychiatric service for mental handicap.

Most mentally handicapped people have the same health care needs as the rest of the population, but some conditions are prone to the development of specific illnesses, such as thyroid dysfunction in people with Down's syndrome. The mentally handicapped seem more prone to developing psychiatric disturbance (with an incidence as high as 50–60%). As longevity is increasing in the mentally handicapped, special problems are being found in the elderly, such as an increased risk of fractures. Special provision must be made, such as respite care facilities, special education, adult training centres, special education (resource) centres, advocates and brokers, and specialist health services to meet special needs, on top of the primary-care services.

Can incidence be reduced?

A third of cases have no known cause. The remaining two-thirds could be reduced by the following measures:

(a) genetic counselling
(b) screening for inherited disorders (including infections)
(c) vaccination, where available, for congenital infections
(d) health education directed at young women, concerning nutrition, smoking, and alcohol consumption during pregnancy
(e) control of exposure of parents/foetus to toxins (eg proposed link between men exposed to hydrocarbons and offspring with Prader-Willi syndrome)
(f) avoid hazards of birth process and improved neonatal care, especially of low- and very-low-birthweight babies
(g) measures to reduce brain-damaging accidents in childhood.

Reducing the incidence of mental illness in the mentally handicapped is the same as for mental illness generally.

Can relapse and readmission rates be reduced?

The early detection of mental illness in the severely mentally handicapped requires special skills because of the communication problems. Prompt management reduces the likelihood of secondary handicaps and the need for admission.

Can total disability be reduced?

Total disability can be reduced by the following measures:

(a) detection of metabolic disorders in infancy, with prompt and adequate treatment of detected cases, to prevent the onset of mental handicap or reduce its impact
(b) detection and appropriate treatment of serious physical illness at an early stage

(c) early detection of sensory defects
(d) early and continuing appropriate remedial education, not necessarily ending at 16
(e) fostering self-help and independence and preventing institutionalisation
(f) providing adequate and appropriate day-care facilities
(g) support for carers
(h) regular monitoring of nutritional status, including minerals and vitamins, and care in the prescribing of psychotropic drugs in the elderly mentally handicapped, to minimise fractures.

Is there an avoidable mortality?

The fact that longevity is increasing in the mentally handicapped is proof that there is avoidable mortality. One continuing problem in the elderly mentally handicapped is respiratory-tract infections and, although deaths from status epilepticus have decreased, deaths due to carcinoma (particularly gastrointestinal), myocardial infarction, and cerebrovascular accident have increased (Jancar, 1988). Improved mortality is due to new antibiotics and anticonvulsants, better diet and care and better environment (Jancar, 1988).

Objectives

These would include:
(a) to ensure all people with a mental handicap receive the same health care as the rest of the population
(b) to ensure that additional special needs receive appropriate services
(c) to ensure that the incidence of mental handicap is reduced
(d) to ensure that prompt detection and appropriate management of serious physical or mental illness occurs to avoid hospital admission or readmission
(e) to ensure that additional disability is prevented
(f) to continue, through research, to prevent avoidable early death
(g) to improve self-esteem and reduce psychiatric morbidity by encouraging improved education attainments and social skills training
(h) to care for the carers, to enable them to continue to care.

Input indicators

These would include:
(a) to foster the widespread establishment of mental handicap registers
(b) to establish enrolment of each person with a mental handicap on the list of a GP
(c) to ensure each DHA has a written policy on the health care provision for the mentally handicapped, including specialist services to meet special needs such as medical and nursing psychiatric care, speech therapy (now in drastically short supply), physiotherapy, occupational therapy–including medical audit
(d) regular assessment of sight and hearing
(e) genetic counselling and continued research in genetics
(f) screening for inherited disorders
(g) vaccination availability and improve uptake
(h) health education, including accident prevention, effects of alcohol and nicotine in pregnancy, etc.
(i) control of environmental hazards
(j) high standards of obstetric and neonatal care

(k) continued research into the special needs of the elderly mentally handicapped
(l) regular monitoring of minerals and vitamins in the elderly mentally handicapped
(m) to ensure appropriate day-care facilities are available, and to improve on work opportunities
(n) to continue the programme of community care to provide as normal a living environment as possible
(o) to improve educational services to help a person reach optimum ability
(p) availability of respite care services to lighten the burden on carers.

Process indicators

Indicators of activity on all the input indicators, including research on how to identify consumer satisfaction, would be required.

Outcome indicators

These would include:
(a) prevalence figures for males and females, for mild/moderate and severe mental handicap, for specific syndromes, and the total
(b) statistics on brain-damaged children left mentally handicapped
(c) statistics on the age at death for men and women as well as the cause of death
(d) hospital admission and readmission rates
(e) statistics on additional handicaps such as sensory defects, behaviour disturbance, motor disability
(f) levels of obtained employment, uptake of day services
(g) improved uptake of respite care services
(h) estimates of consumer satisfaction (possibly by questionnaires)
(i) a record of the registers available nationally.

Alcohol misuse

The incidence depends on the definition of what constitutes misuse. For example, 6% men and 1% women are very heavy drinkers, while 25% men and 9% women are drinking more than agreed 'sensible' levels. The consequences of alcohol misuse may be physical, psychological and social, and arise both from chronic alcohol misuse (eg cirrhosis) and from acute intoxication (eg road accidents).

Can incidence be reduced?

The incidence of alcohol misuse can be reduced by a wide range of factors which influence either availability or demand.

Can relapse rate and hospital readmission rates be reduced?

Relapse rates and readmission rates can be reduced. The best chance of success is when the problem drinking is at an early stage. Minimal intervention (simple advice, brief follow-up, and feed-back on progress) has a high rate of success at this stage, particularly if the family can be involved. Improvement is much lower for severe chronic drinking problems.

Can total disability be reduced?

While some of the pathological changes caused by excessive alcohol consumption are irreversible, a remarkable degree of physiological recovery can occur with abstinence and attention to nutrition and vitamins. Problem drinkers may have special accommodation needs, require medical treatment to prevent further physical disability or continued support to stop or reduce drinking.

Is there an avoidable mortality?

Alcohol-related accidents and illness cause around 7,000 deaths each year and 15% of alcoholics commit suicide.

Objectives

These would include:
- (a) to reduce the prevalence of alcohol misuse
- (b) to reduce relapse and readmission rates with alcohol-related diagnoses
- (c) to reduce suicide rates
- (d) to reduce premature mortality, especially from chronic liver disease
- (e) to eradicate or reduce homelessness among people who misuse alcohol.

Input indicators

These would be:
- (a) education and support for primary-care teams to encourage screening, detection and better management of problem drinkers
- (b) continuing education of primary- and secondary-care teams about assessment of suicide
- (c) provision of a range of services including advice centres, day centres, detoxification facilities (home and residential), hostel accommodation, hospital-based services, and community-based services (eg community alcohol team)
- (d) case register.

Outcome indicators

These would be:
- (a) hospital admissions, discharges and deaths with a diagnosis of alcohol-related mental illness or liver disease
- (b) local alcohol consumption-level and pattern (obtainable by community survey)
- (c) prevalence of suicide in local patients with alcohol misuse
- (d) prevalence figures from local case register.

Drug misuse

The absolute number of drug misusers is unknown. It has been estimated that nationally there are 75,000–100,000 misusers of opiate drugs, and as many again who misuse a variety of other illicit drugs (Department of Health and Social Security, 1988, 1989). This estimate excludes cannabis users (possibly three million nationally).

Research has suggested that over ten years, 40% of illicit opiate users will become abstinent, one-third will achieve greater social stability, and the remainder will continue chaotic use or die. There is an annual mortality of 200–300. Illicit drug users have high rates of accident, and accidental overdose. Injecting drug use with shared injecting equipment is associated with 3% of reported AIDS cases nationally, and an increasing proportion of reported HIV-infected people (currently 10%) (Director of Public Health Laboratory Service, 1990). Social and relationship problems are common, and in some areas there is well researched association with unemployment and homelessness. Drug-related legal problems further disadvantage the user. Management of the problematic drug user must therefore contain not only psychiatric but medical and social elements of care.

Can incidence be reduced?

Law enforcement has a major role in reducing the availability of illicit drugs. Health education on the effects of drugs, and the appropriate use of medication, can improve information about their use or misuse, but there is no clear evidence in the international research literature that drug education necessarily has any long-term effect on illicit drug taking. There is, however, some recent evidence that information and education about the HIV-related risks of sharing needles may influence people (Stimson *et al*, 1988). Benzodiazepine dependence can be reduced by careful assessment and prescribing. The illicit misuse of other pharmaceutical drugs can be reduced by good security in the storage and careful prescribing of controlled drugs.

Can relapse rates and readmission rates be reduced?

Early intervention and harm-minimisation strategies can reduce physical morbidity and legal involvement. Habilitative strategies particularly for young adolescent users, including opportunities for education, training and employment, may reduce continued misuse and relapse (d'Orban, 1982). For chronic users, similar rehabilitative strategies, and the provision of adequate housing, can improve stability, and provide a basis for appropriate domiciliary care should HIV infection supervene.

Can total disability be reduced?

Provision of adequate rehabilitative services and long-term support can improve social and health functioning, even in the absence of abstinence.

Is there an avoidable mortality?

Drug users may lack access to primary health care, leading to unnecessary morbidity and mortality from usually non-fatal conditions. In chronic users immunosuppression related to drug use *per se* and to injecting has been demonstrated. Health education about the risks of shared injecting may reduce the risks of HIV infection and hepatitis B. Drug users following involuntary withdrawal (as in prison) are at higher risk of death from accidental overdose, due to loss of tolerance following release. Clear information and health education before release are necessary. Controlled substitution prescribing reduces the risk of mortality from use of illicit, contaminated drugs.

Objectives

These would include:

(a) to reduce the incidence of prescribed problematic drug use
(b) to reduce relapse rates and readmissions
(c) to reduce deterioration in social functioning
(d) to reduce the rate of accidental overdose and infections (including HIV)
(e) to reduce mortality
(f) to reduce overall health morbidity

(g) to reduce unemployment
(h) to reduce inadequate housing

Input indicators

These would be:
(a) accessible and available primary care services
(b) community-based specialist drug agencies providing a range of treatment options
(c) designated secondary-level hospital provision
(d) systems of social support to users and their families
(e) appropriate health education for users and their families
(f) adequate rehabilitation services, including hostels, half-way houses, and housing
(g) specific harm-minimisation strategies, needle-exchange projects, outreach work
(h) adequate training, education and employment opportunities
(i) training for all professionals likely to make contact with drug users.

Process indicators

These would be indicators of activity on all the above factors.

Outcome indicators

These would include:
(a) incidence of prevalence data from the regional drug database and the Home Office Addicts Index, supplemented by local-community research surveys
(b) hospital admission and readmission rates for all drug-related conditions
(c) attendances at designated day centres
(d) contacts with community psychiatric nurses
(e) employment rates of drug users
(f) prevalence of HIV and hepatitis B in injecting drug users, their sexual partners and children
(g) local drug-related offence rate
(h) coroner's records of accidental overdose.

Conclusion

At present, most data from the Department of Health are gathered on indicators of process. As financial resources are at such a premium, it would seem more useful to concentrate them on measuring inputs and outcomes first of all, and only to use process where necessary, to investigate shortfalls in achieving desired objectives.

The suggestions for health indicators here are not in any way intended to be exhaustive, but rather to serve as pointers towards the kind of measurement which clinicians, researchers, health authorities, family practitioner committees and DPHs can usefully engage in to fulfil their objectives of assessing quality of health care. There are opportunities for collaboration between secondary-care services and DPHs (referred to earlier), and also between primary-care and secondary-care services. For example, GPs, as part of their new contract, are required to screen patients over 75 annually. Such a screen should properly include scales for dementia and depression, and therefore collaboration with the secondary-care services before and after data collection would be mutually beneficial.

Acknowledgements

I am greatly indebted to my colleagues Dr D Black, Dr D Brooksbank, Dr D Jones, Dr H Markowe, Dr P Mason, Dr J Reed and Dr J Shanks and Mr R Anderson at the Department of Health for helpful advice on earlier versions of this manuscript, and Miss Lynette Timms for secretarial assistance.

References

Bennett, D H. (1982) Management and rehabilitation of affective psychoses. In *Handbook of Psychiatry, vol. 3, Psychoses of Uncertain Aetiology* (eds J K Wing & L Wing). Cambridge: Cambridge University Press.

Bergner, M, Bobbit, R A, Kressel, S, *et al* (1979) The sickness impact profile: conceptual formulation and methodology for the development of a health status measure. In *Sociomedical Health Indicators* (eds J Elinson & A E Siegmann). New York: Baywood.

Bergner, M, Kaplan, R M & Ware, J E (1987) Evaluating health measures. Commentary: measuring overall health: an evaluation of three important approaches. *Journal of Chronic Diseases,* **40** (suppl.), 235–265

Berkman, P (1975) Survival and a modicum of indulgence in the sick role. *Medical Care*, **13**, 85.

Bice, T W (1979) Comments on health indicators. Methodological perspectives. In *Sociomedical Health Indicators* (eds J Elinson & A E Siegmann). New York: Baywood.

Birchwood, M., Smith, J., Macmillan, S., *et al* (1989) Predicting relapse in schizophrenia: the development and implementation of an early signs monitoring system using patients and families as observers. *Psychological Medicine,* **19**, 649–656.

Brewin, C R., Wing, J K., Mangin, S P., *et al* (1987) Principles and practice of measuring needs in the longterm mentally ill; the MRC Needs for Care Assessment. *Psychological Medicine,* **17**, 971–981.

Brewin, C R., Wing, J K., Mangin, S P., *et al* (1988) Needs for care-the longterm mentally ill; a report from the Camberwell High Contact Survey. *Psychological Medicine,* **18**, 457–468.

Bucher, H & Gutzwiller, F (1988) Evaluating an indicator of preventive health behaviour derived from a national study. *Health Promotion,* **3**, 73–78.

Carr, W & Wolfe, S (1979) Unmet needs as social indicators. In *Sociomedical Health Indicators* (eds J Elinson & A E Siegmann). New York: Baywood.

Cook, T D & Campbell, D T (1976) The design and conduct of quasi experiments and true experiments in field settings. In *Handbook of Industrial and Organisational Psychology* (ed. M D Dunnette). Chicago: Rand McNally.

Cooper, A F (1976) Deafness and psychiatric illness. *British Journal of Psychiatry,* **129**, 216–226.

Corbett, J A (1979) Psychiatric morbidity and mental retardation. In *Psychiatric Illness and Mental Handicap* (eds F E James & R P Snaith). London: Gaskell.

Culver, A J (1983) *Health Indicators. An International Study for the European Science Foundation*. Oxford: Martin Robertson.

Cutting, J (1985) *The Psychology of Schizophrenia.* Edinburgh: Churchill Livingstone.

Day, K (1983) A hospital based psychiatric unit for mentally handicapped adults. *Mental Handicap,* **11**, 137–140.

Dean, K (1988) Issues in the development of health promotion indicators. *Health Promotion,* **3**, 13–21.

Dell, S & Gibbens, T C N (1971) Remands of women offenders for medical reports. *Medicine, Science and the Law,* **11**, 117–127.

Department of Health and Social Security (1988) *On the State of the Public Health for the Year 1987.* London: HMSO.

Department of Health and Social Security (1988) *Aids and Drug Misuse Part I. Report by the Advisory Council on the Misuse of Drugs.* London: HMSO.

Department of Health and Social Security (1989) *Aids and Drug Misuse Part II. Report by the Advisory Council on the Misuse of Drugs.* London: HMSO.

Director of the Public Health Laboratory Service (1990) Acquired immune deficiency syndrome in England and Wales to end 1993; projections using data to end September 1989. *Communicable Disease Report, January 1990.* London: Public Health Laboratory Service.

D'Orban, P (1982) Drug dependence. In *Handbook of Psychiatry, vol. 4 The Neuroses and Personality Disorders.* (eds G F M Russell & L A Hersov). Cambridge: Cambridge University Press.

Earls, F & Jung, K G (1987) Temperament and home environment characteristics as causal factors in the early development of childhood psychopathology, *Journal of the American Academy of Child and Adolescent Psychiatry,* **26**, 491–498.

Falloon, I R H, Boyd, J L, McGill, C W, *et al* (1982) Family management in the prevention of exacerbations of schizophrenia. *New England Journal of Medicine,* **306**, 1437–1440.

Falloon, I R H, Boyd, J L, McGill, C W, *et al* (1985) Family management in the prevention of morbidity of schizophrenia: clinical outcome of a two year longitudinal study. *Archives of General Psychiatry,* **42**, 887–896.

Fox, A J & Goldblatt, P O (1982) *Longitudinal Study–Sociodemographic Morality Differential,* LS No. 1, 1971–1975. London: HMSO.

Goldberg, D (1978) *Manual of the General Health Questionnaire.* Windsor: NFER.

Goldberg, D & Huxley, P (1980) *Mental Illness in the Community: The Pathway to Psychiatric Care.* London: Tavistock.

Gulbinat, W (1983) Mental health problem assessment and information support direction of WHO's work. *World Health Statistics Quarterly,* **36**, 224–233.

Gunn, J, Robertson, G, Dell, S, *et al* (1978) *Psychiatric Aspects of Imprisonment*. London: Academic Press.

Hansluwka, H E (1985) Measuring the health of populations, indicators and interpretations. *Social Science and Medicine,* **20**, 1207–1224.

Hawton, K (1987) Assessment of suicide risk. *British Journal of Psychiatry,* **150**, 145–153.

Hunt, S M (1988) Subjective health indicators and health promotion. *Health Promotion,* **3**, 23–24.

Hyde, C, Bridges, K, Goldberg, D *et al* (1987) Evaluation of a hostel ward. A controlled study using modified cost benefit analysis. *British Journal of Psychiatry,* **151**, 805–812.

Jancar, J (1988) Consequences of longer life for the mentally handicapped. *Geriatric Medicine,* **18**, 81–87.

Jenkins, R (1985) Sex differences in minor psychiatric morbidity. *Psychological Medicine* (monograph suppl. 7).

Johnstone, A & Goldberg, D (1966) Psychiatric screening in general practice. *Lancet, i,* 605–608.

Kolvin, I, Miller, F J W, Scott, D M, *et al* (1990) Continuities of deprivation? The Newcastle 1,000 family study. ESRC/DHSS. *Studies in Deprivation and Disadvantage,* **15**, 379–393.

Leff, J, Kuipers, L, Berkowitz, R, *et al* (1985) A controlled trial of social intervention in the families of schizophrenia patients: two-year follow up. *British Journal of Psychiatry,* **146**, 594–600.

Lohr, K N & Ware, J E, Jr (eds) (1987) Proceedings of the advances in health assessment conference. *Journal of Chronic Diseases,* **40**, (suppl. 1).

McDowell, I & Newell, C (1987) *Measuring Health: A Guide to Rating Scales and Questionnaires.* Oxford: Oxford University Press.

Miles, C P (1977) Conditions predisposing to suicide: a review, *Journal of Nervous and Mental Disease,* **164**, 231–246.

Mootz, M (1988) Health (promotion) indicators; realistic and unrealistic expectations. *Health Promotion,* **3**, 79–84.

Newton, J (1988) Approaches to prevention: supporting troubled persons. In *Preventing Mental Illness.* London: Routledge & Kegan Paul.

Noack, H & McQueen, D (1988) Towards health promotion indicators. *Health Promotion,* **3**, 73–78.

Patrick, D & Erickson, P (1987) *Assessing Health Related Quality of Life in General Population Surveys: Issues and Recommendations.* Washington, DC: National Center for Health Statistics.

Rainer, J D (1982) Genetics of schizophrenia. In *Handbook of Psychiatry, vol. 3. Psychoses of Uncertain Aetiology* (eds J K Wing & L Wing). Cambridge University Press.

Reich, T, Claninger, C R, Suarez, B, *et al* (1982) Genetics of the affective psychoses. In *Handbook of Psychiatry, vol. 3. Psychoses of Uncertain Aetiology* (eds J K Wing & L Wing). Cambridge: Cambridge University Press.

Reveley, A (1985) Genetic counselling for schizophrenia. *British Journal of Psychiatry,* **147**, 107–112.

Rosenthal, D (1971) *Genetics of Psychopathology*. New York: McGraw Hill.

Rutter, M (1989) Isle of Wight revisited: twenty-five years of child psychiatric epidemiology. *Journal of the American Academy of Child and Adolescent Psychiatry,* **28**, 633–653.

Rutter, M, Graham, P & Yule, W (1970*a*) *A Neuropsychiatric Study in Childhood*. London: SIMP/Heinemann.

Rutter, M, Tizard, J & Whitemore, K, (eds) (1970*b*) *Education, Health and Behaviour*. London: Longman.

Rutter, M & Giller, H (1983) *Juvenile Delinquency-Trends and Perspectives*. Harmondsworth: Penguin.

Sainsbury, P (1983) Validity and reliability of trends in suicide statistics. *World Health Statistics Quarterly,* **36**, 339–348.

Shaw, C D (1989) Audit in internal medicine. *British Journal of Hospital Medicine,* **42**, 19.

Siegmann, A E (1979) A classification of sociomedical health indicators: perspectives for health administrators and health planners. In *Sociomedical Health Indicators* (eds J Elinson & A E Siegmann). New York: Baywood.

Sims, A & Prior, P (1978) The pattern of mortality in severe neuroses. *British Journal of Psychiatry,* **133**, 299–305.

Stimson, G V, Alldritt, L, Dolan, K, *et al* (1988) *Injecting Equipment Exchange Schemes: Final Report*. London: Goldsmith's College.

Thompson, C (ed.) (1989) *The Instruments of Psychiatric Research*. Chichester: Wiley.

Torgensen, S (1983) Genetics of neuroses: the effects of sampling variation upon the twin concordance ratio. *British Journal of Psychiatry,* **142**, 126–132.

West, D J & Farrington, D P (1977) *The Delinquent Way of Life*. London: Heinemann Educational.

Wing, J (1982) Rehabilitation and management of schizophrenia. In *Handbook of Psychiatry, vol. 3. Psychoses of Uncertain Aetiology*. (eds J K Wing & L Wing). Cambridge: Cambridge University Press.

World Health Organisation (1948) *Official Records of the World Health Organization, No. 2,* pp. 100. Geneva: WHO.

World Health Organisation (1981) *Development of Indicators for Monitoring Progress Towards Health for All by the Year 2000*. Geneva: WHO.

Wilson, R (1981) Do health indicators indicate health? *American Journal of Public Health,* **71**, 461.

Audit in Mental Health

Professor John Wing

Abstract

The task of audit in mental health is discussed under four headings.

1. Mental disorders are characterized by psychological as well as physical dysfunctions. Because the dysfunctions are often persistent, many disorders should be described in terms of handicap as well as of illness. The psychological dysfunctions are often 'invisible' and not measurable using physical investigations. These characteristics are not unique to psychological medicine but they do need to be recognized when discussing audit and particularly when measuring outcomes.

2. The audit strategy of the Royal College of Psychiatrists at a time when responsibility for 'community care' is being divided between statutory authorities, is briefly described. A Clinical Audit Section is being set up in the College Research Unit; its priorities are considered.

3. The value of good quality statistical data concerning the sociodemographic and service profiles of health and local authorities, and the limitations of the Korner minimum dataset in this respect, are emphasized, and illustrated by data describing the rundown of the large hospitals and the partial build up of alternatives. The motivation of clinical teams to contribute to the collection of high quality data is discussed.

4. Technical problems involved in measuring 'mental health' outcomes are described and some solutions discussed.

Introduction

I propose to discuss the concept and practice of audit from the point of view of someone whose research has been concerned mainly with themes that are covered broadly by the now old-fashioned, but still I hope respectable, term 'social medicine'. Only recently, while setting up a new Research Unit for the Royal College of Psychiatrists, have I come across the term 'audit' applied to many of these same themes. Like David Mechanic, a medical sociologist attending a conference on psychiatric epidemiology in 1969, who found that he had been an epidemiologist all his professional life (Mechanic, 1970), I have discovered that part of what I have been doing can be redefined as audit. It is an interesting part because it is concerned with 'state of the art' medical practice-how this is defined, how it can be implemented, and how the effects can be evaluated.

Many research workers tend, for good reasons, to avoid becoming too much involved in promoting the application of their results. They feel that others should evaluate their work in a broader context and decide what to incorporate into practice and what to leave out. This is a slow and somewhat chancy process; 'best practice' is not always chosen or, if chosen, practised. Audit, on the other hand, depends on self-evaluation on the part of individuals and groups involved in clinical work, using criteria that are necessarily imperfect but which can be used to appraise everyday decisions, with the stated aim of improving practice.

There is much to be said for caution but research workers could make much greater efforts to present their results in a 'user friendly' form. That means frank consideration of the cons as well as the pros. One answer to the question, 'Who should audit the auditors?', is that the designs and techniques and the mandatory public scrutiny which are a routine part of the scientific process, should also be applied to the implementation of results, to determine whether audit activities actually change practice for the better.

The advantages of such an approach can be illustrated by discussing it from four points of view: first, a consideration of the special problems that arise when auditing practices relating to mental health problems; second, a brief description of how our College is beginning to tackle its responsibilities for audit; third, a discussion of a specific example of a problem central to the planning of mental health services, using available statistical data; finally, a discussion of how 'bottom-up' audit activities and measurement of outcomes can influence 'top-down' planning procedures.

It will not be possible to deal in any detail with the audit of mental health issues that arise mainly in primary care or outside the National Health Service altogether, important though these are. I should also say that all the opinions expressed are my own.

Models for audit in mental health

The range of mental disorders is illustrated by Chapter F of the tenth International Classification of Diseases (ICD10), about to be published by the World Health Organization. Each category contains disorders that may be expressed in mild to extremely severe forms, which may be transitory or persistent. Because of time and space constraints, I shall have to limit comment to the more severe disorders, those most likely to lead to referral to specialist services, but these do include examples of all the categories listed.

Although there are plenty of exceptions, mental disorders tend, on the whole, to be recurrent or chronic. Apart from dementia, most occur during the productive years of life. A model of audit similar to one for diabetes mellitus, in which concepts of disability are as important as concepts of disease, is therefore appropriate.

Terminology is important here. The term 'mental handicap', for example, which is the official UK substitute for WHO's 'mental retardation', causes endless confusion because schizophrenia can only be called an illness, although it is often associated with severe disability. Because the psychological dysfunctions causing a degree of social disablement are 'invisible' (and, unlike diabetes, usually cannot be demonstrated by physical investigations) they can easily be ignored or denied.

The Commons Social Services Committee, in its two reports on community care for people with mental disorders (1985; 1990), has avoided this trap by always referring to 'mental disability'. Members have thus also grasped the essential point that community care for the mentally disabled requires the provision of methods of care that involve at the same time both health and social types of expertise. Health Authorities are charged with the responsibility for providing 'health care' to people for whom Social Services Departments (with very different philosophies, resources and priorities) are providing 'social care' and *vice versa* (Flynn and Common, 1990; Wistow, 1990). The Committee's minutes of evidence from the Royal College of Nursing illustrates the problem. Reference is made to

Table 1 The range of mental disorders

International Classification of Diseases, 10th Revision

Examples from Chapter F: Mental and Behavioural Disorders, including Disorders of Psychological Development

F0. Organic mental disorders, eg
- F00-F03 Dementias
- F04 Organic amnesic syndromes
- F05 Delirium

F1. Mental disorders due to use of psychoactive substances, eg
- F10 Alcohol
- F11 Opiods
- F12 Cannabinoids

F2. Psychoses eg
- F20 Schizophrenias
- F22 Persistent delusional disorders
- F25 Schizoaffective disorders

F3. Affective disorders, eg
- F30 Manic episodes
- F31 Bipolar affective disorder
- F32 Depressive episode

F4. Neurotic, stress-related and somatoform disorders, eg
- F40 Phobic anxiety disorders
- F41 Generalized anxiety disorder
- F42 Obsessive-compulsive disorder
- F43 Stress and adjustment disorders
- F44 Dissociative disorders
- F45 Somatoform disorders

F5. Behavioural syndromes associated with physiological disturbances and physical factors, eg
- F50 Eating disorders
- F51 Sleep disorders
- F52 Sexual dysfunction

F6. Disorders of adult personality and behaviour, eg
- F60 Specific personality disorders

F7. Mental retardation

F8. Disorders of psychological development, eg
- F80 Disorders of speech and language
- F84 Includes autism and Asperger's syndrome

F9. Disorders with an onset in childhood

the distinction between a 'health' bath and a 'social' bath, which depends not on the reason for needing help but on what kind of professional provides it.

These are matters that public health physicians have to understand because service planning must take account of them. General practitioners, with their very broad spectrum of care, and those involved with the care of people with physical disabilities, also cannot evade the problems that arise. Psychiatrists, willy-nilly, work at the heart of this complexity at a time when many large mental hospitals are closing or are moribund and responsibility for community alternatives is precariously and ambiguously divided between agencies that sometimes seem to be competing rather than cooperating.

The implications for audit are perhaps less well understood, though it is pleasing to note that 'medical audit' is now sometimes replaced by the broader 'clinical audit'. I will use the latter term as a code to signal the fact that audit in mental health has to be judged by the reduction of social disablement, not just by the reduction of physical disability.

Because this entails a consideration of social disadvantage and adverse self and social attitudes (particularly to mental disability), this has the added attraction of ensuring that quality of life is added to quality of care as one of the central aims of audit. It is on the other side of the same coin as disablement (Wing, 1990a).

A strategy for audit in mental health

The aim of our College's audit strategy, in the longer term, is to improve the quality of patient care through the scrutiny of routinely collected information about clinical work and services, and ongoing peer review and educational activities, which eventully become part of ordinary clinical practice and provide clinicians as well as managers with information relevant to administration and planning.

More specifically, the College aims, with the help of a dedicated Clinical Audit Section of the Research Unit, to provide:

(a) recommendations concerning standards of clinical record keeping;
(b) methods of registering data that are both user-friendly and relevant to monitoring the quality of care in a local District;
(c) guidelines on the minimum structure of services required by each sub-specialty, with advice on recognising the epidemiological characteristics of higher and lower need districts;
(d) agreed clinical standards in some areas of particular public or clinical concern, for example because of high social or financial costs or a high public profile, or because they are very common or particularly severe or chronic;
(e) a central literature and information base, and an advisory centre, for those who wish to undertake audit locally.

Some of the priority areas for the construction or updating of guidelines include:

(a) the most effective and economic use of short-term hospital care;
(b) * assessment and prescription of health and social care for vulnerable people after discharge from hospital (College, 1989);
(c) * best documented practice in prescribing medication as part of the long term care of people with schizophrenia or bipolar disorders;
(d) * the use of electroplexy;
(e) * the use of the Mental Health Act;
(f) scrutiny of suicide rates;
(g) psychiatric care for people with a mental handicap;
(h) the care of mentally disabled people who are living in accommodation for the homeless or actually on the streets;
(i) information booklets for patients and carers;
(j) the construction of guidelines for effective inter-professional working.

*Guidelines exist for items marked with an asterisk, but these may not be observed in practice. They may need updating, or may need drawing to the attention of College members.

The achievement of these aims will be facilitated by the information generated by the Clinical Audit Section of the Research Unit, headed by a senior consultant psychiatrist, assisted by a senior registrar and advised by experts in public health medicine, computer technology and health economics. The College Research Unit provides an appropriate working environment because several of the research studies being planned or undertaken have similar aims, although the time scale is longer and the designs and methodology more complex. The fact that the Unit is part of the College but is seen as supplying independent and, if necessary, critical advice on the basis of the results of its studies, will be a major advantage. There will also be a productive interaction, since some of the audit projects are likely to provide a sampling frame and initial data base for more intensive evaluative studies by the research staff.

It will be most economical to discuss the technical problems of audit from two points of view. The first is 'top down', in the sense that the data is not collected directly by clinicians in the course of their work but represent statistical abstractions. The second is 'bottom up'.

Mental health information systems

The decline in the resident population of mental illness hospitals since the peak of bed occupancy in 1954 has been well documented, though the change to Korner has led to a recent hiatus. In general, the decline has been chiefly noticeable in the group of very long stay residents (ie over 5 years), where it has been due largely to deaths, except in those instances, such as Powick (Brockington and Hall, 1990, in press), or Darenth Park in the case of mental handicap (Korman and Glennester, 1989; L Wing, 1990), where special efforts have been made to close hospitals. The rate of occupancy for those residing less than a year (about 60 per 100,000 in English hospitals) has not much changed. More significantly, nor have the rates for those staying between 1 and 5 years (about 40 per 100,000).

In a little known paper for regional statisticians, Graham Robertson (1981) calculated that by the end of 1991, there would be 140 in-patients per 100,000 inhabitants in an average Health District, 80 of whom would be long-stay (resident for more than a year). If those with a diagnosis of dementia are omitted, there would be just over 50 short-stay and 50 long-stay in-patients per 100,000 population. This estimate assumed no substantial changes in service practice. Of course, there have been such changes. However, the question arises as to how far the projected rates can be used to estimate the numbers needing high-dependency care in some form of sheltered accommodation, whatever this may be called (Wing, 1986; 1990b).

This is a key question for audit but it cannot be answered by data from the Mental Health Enquiry, nor by the Korner dataset. Eight Psychiatric Case Registers used to produce good quality data for their local Districts, which varied substantially in their characteristics. One of the most striking differences was the change in population size over time. Oxford, for example, doubled its population between 1921 and 1981. Middle-sized industrial cities like Cardiff, Nottingham and Southampton stayed more or less at the national average, while the population of Camberwell was cut by half.

The number of occupied beds in the three length-of-stay categories, and the rates of 'new long-stay' accumulation, were closely associated with local population dynamics and socio-economic indices (Wing, 1989). The correlation between recruitment rates (1–2 years in hospital, age under 65) and the Jarman index of deprivation was 0.76. Graham Thornicroft (personal communication) has made the same calculation, using data from the Health Districts within the catchment area served by two other hospitals due for closure (Friern and Claybury), with a virtually identical result.

The Jarman index can be unpacked. The important components, apart from age and sex, are poverty, social isolation and ethnicity; social isolation probably being the most important so far as admission rates are concerned. Note should also be taken of the effects of positive against negative migration, factors affecting access to care facilities (topography, public transport, travel expense, etc.), and local traditions established by earlier 'product champions'.

Mention of Darenth, Friern and Powick hospitals is a reminder that all of them have been the subject of health services research. In the case of Friern and Claybury, the research unit (TAPS) is supported by the NE Thames Regional Health Authority, with contributions from the Department of Health and charitable foundations. Combining top-down and bottom-up approaches in this way allows the planner to gain the best from both worlds. Most Districts, however, cannot afford the luxury of their own research unit. It is nevertheless possible to gather good quality local information. This forms the subject of my last section.

Outcome indicators and the assessment of need

One advantage of a College Research Unit is that it can use its facilities and expertise to adapt techniques that were designed for complex data collection so as to make them user-friendly. It is not sufficient to tell clinicians that using such methods will provide them with information that will help them take part in formulating plans for their local services, instead of standing helplessly by while others make the decisions. That is true but it is not enough. There has to be a more direct reward. The CRISP system devised by Dr Peter Rohde and now being developed at Riverside bids fair to pass this test.

Our Research Unit is engaged in developing techniques for studying one of the problems of highest priority for the College, and for psychiatry more generally: how to combine the most effective use of scarce short-stay hospital places with adequate long-term community support for those who need it.

The plan is to collect detailed information about a period prevalence sample of people admitted to hospital from two privileged and two deprived Health Districts. The research instrument, which has already been piloted, contains sections on the social and clinical problems causing admission, the facilities that might have been used to prevent admission if they had been available, anticipated vulnerability to readmission, and discharge plans. This last section is based on College guidance for good practice. The data will be analysed in conjunction with a structural and a sociodemographic profile for each District. Data is entered directly to a laptop computer file, and can be processed at once according to a predetermined programme to yield individual profiles and group tables.

The results will be of immediate interest to clinicians and managers, showing what the local problems are and how they compare with those of contrasting Districts. The research experience can also be used to simplify the technique, which will then be used on a wider scale.

Another advantage is that the exercise will provide a sampling frame for a one year follow-up needs assessment study, including all patients thought to be vulnerable and a sample of the rest. The needs assessment system was designed originally for long-term attenders at day hospitals and centres (Brewin et al, 1987, 1988; Brewin and Wing, 1988; Brugha et al, 1988). It was designed (though not consciously) according to the three parts of the classical audit strategy–assessment of problems (potential needs), prescription of help specific to each problem identified (needs for care, for caring agents, and for settings in which the care should be given), and follow-up to discover whether unmet needs are met (outcomes).

The results will take longer to make available but, because of the known sampling frames and known local sociodemographic and service profiles, comparisons between Districts will be enlightening.

It will be of great potential value for the Clinical Audit Group, concerned with more 'hands on' audit activities, to interact in the Research Unit with workers carrying out more intensive studies. This will facilitate the adaptation of the admission audit and the needs assessment techniques for a variety of circumstances and clientele. Both have been implemented for lap computer by Dr Gyles Glover. Together they could form a basis for 'bottom up' mini-registers that would not only be friendly in the sense that they would provide case summaries, discharge letters, routine statistics, and performance indicators for clinical teams, but would form a basis for a much deeper kind of 'bottom-up' audit of on-going clinical activities.

The College is well placed to sponsor this kind of research and help the implementation of results that are seen by members as helpful to themselves and their patients. Specialist Sections of the College will wish to promote such studies across the whole range of mental disorders and service problems. ICD10, which has operationalized Diagnostic Criteria for Research (DCR), will help to resolve part of a problem that has long bedevilled psychiatric research. The tenth edition of the Present State Examination, part of a set of schedules known as SCAN, is accompanied by software that will process PSE10 and other data according to the DCR rules (Wing et al, 1990).

Conclusions

Although some Colleges are ahead of us, partly because the problems of audit are more strictly 'medical' than those discussed so far, we aim to make our methods of assessment and measurement no less stringent relative to the difficulty of the task. Together with the other audit projects described in this publication, we can make a strong bid to improve the average level of clinical care and also to evaluate its success.

References

Brewin C, Wing J K, Mangen S, Brugha T S and MacCarthy B (1987) Principles and practice of measuring needs in the long-term mentally ill. Psychological Medicine 17: 971–981.

Brewin C and Wing J K (1988) The MRC Needs for Care Assessment manual. MRC Social Psychiatry Unit.

Brewin C R, Wing J K, Mangen S, Brugha T S, MacCarthy B and Lesage A (1988) Needs for care among the long-term mentally ill: A report from the Camberwell High Contact Survey. Psychological Medicine 18: 457–468.

Brugha T S, Wing J K, Brewin C R, MacCarthy B, Mangen S, Lesage A and Mumford J (1988) The problems of people in long-term psychiatric day care. An introduction to the Camberwell High Contact Survey. Psychological Medicine 18: 443–456.

Brockington I and Hall P (eds) (1990) The closure of Powick, ch.2, pp. 10–19. London: Gaskell.

Flynn N and Common R (1990) Contracts for community care. DoH commissioned paper, CCI 4.

Korman N and Glennerster H (1990) Hospital closure. A political and economic study. Milton Keynes: Philadelphia.

Mechanic D (1970) Problems and prospects in psychiatric epidemiology. In: Psychiatric epidemiology. (eds) Hare W H and Wing J K. pp. 3–22. London: Oxford University Press.

Mangen S and Brewin C (1990) The measurement of need. In: Bebbington P (ed) Social psychiatry. Theory, methodology and practice. London; Transaction Press.

Robertson G (1981) The provision of inpatient facilities for the mentally ill. A paper to assist NHS planners. Unpublished. DHSS.

Royal College of Psychiatrists (1989) Guidelines for Good Medical Practice in Discharge and Aftercare Procedures.

Social Services Committee, House of Commons (1985) Community care with special reference to adult mentally ill and mentally handicapped. Second report of the Committee. London: HMSO.

Social Services Committee, House of Commons (1990) Community care. Services for people with a mental handicap and with a mental illness. London: HMSO.

Wing J K (1986) The cycle of planning and evaluation. In: Wilkinson G and Freeman H (eds) The provision of mental health services in Britain. The way ahead. London: Gaskell.

Wing J K (ed) (1989) Health service planning and research. Contributions from Psychiatric Case Registers. London: Gaskell.

Wing J K (1990a) Meeting the needs of people with psychiatric disorders. Social Psychiatry and Psychiatric Epidemiology 25: 2–8.

Wing J K (1990b) The functions of asylum. British Journal of Psychiatry 157, pp. 822–827.

Wing J K, Babor T, Brugha T, Burke J, Cooper J, Giel R, Jablensky A, Regier D and Sartorius N (1990) SCAN; Schedules for clinical assessment in neuropsychiatry. Archives of general psychiatry 47: 589–593.

Wing L (1989) Hospital Closure and the Resettlement of Residents. Aldershot: Avebury.

Wistow G (1990) Community care planning: A review of past experience and future imperatives. DoH commissioned paper, CCI 3.

Appendix

The Royal College of Psychiatrists: Preliminary report on Medical Audit

I. Remit of the Working Party from Council

1. To define and distinguish between clinical audit, peer review and performance indicators.
2. To collect information within the general area of audit, appraise what is most useful for measuring performance in psychiatric practice and make proposals for audit that can be subsequently evaluated.
3. To examine ways in which audits of service and individual units are carried out and what variations have been devised to meet local circumstances and requirements.
4. To consider issues to do with management appraisal.

II. Definitions

1. **Medical Audit** can be defined as the systematic, critical analysis of the quality of medical care, including the procedures used for diagnosis and treatment, the use of resources, and the resulting outcome and quality of life for the patients. (Working paper 6, Paragraph 1.1 of the National Health Service Review).

   Throughout its discussions, the Working Group has preferred to use the term 'Clinical Audit' which includes the work of all members of the multidisciplinary team, and which is therefore more appropriate to psychiatry. In addition to the one just given, the following definitions have been made:
2. **Clinical Audit** is the generic term used to cover ways in which evaluation can be for:

   (a) to determine the effectiveness of a specific treatment, a treatment regime, or a treatment setting,

   (b) a random evaluation of run-of-the-mill cases,

   (c) an examination of the occurrence of unusual but undesirable events such as maternal deaths in childbirth, acts of violence, absconding etc.,

   (d) to provide statistics for financial planning and accounting.

   Clinical Audit resembles clinical research in several ways, but is not research as no hypothesis is tested.

   There are two aspects of Clinical Audit: Quantitative and Qualitative. The managerial emphasis has been on measures of quantity (eg as in the Körner data) but the clinicians should give at least equal emphasis to measures of quality.
3. **Peer Review** is a method of Clinical Audit in which the quality of the performance of a particular practitioner is measured by and compared with that of his colleagues.
4. **Performance Indicators** are ratios of output to input. They measure quantity.

   Input measures include: wtes (whole-time equivalents) of consultant time, members of para-medical staff such as psychologists, occupational therapists, etc.

   Output measures include: bed occupancy, numbers of patients seen in a clinic session. Department of Health performance indicators have used Körner recommended minimum data which are found to be unsuitable for those specialists which have moved away from traditional hospital practice, especially child and adolescent psychiatry (Nicol, 1989), the psychiatry of old age (see report of working group) and the psychiatry of mental handicap.

5. **Quality Assurance** is another generic term meaning methods employed to maintain and improve standards. One example of this would be the College's educational approval visits.
6. **Monitoring** is a technique of Clinical Audit whereby there is regular re-assessment of some aspect of the service, eg routine examination of untoward incidents such as suicide, aggression or wandering off under section (see 2(c)).

III. Levels of Audit

1. Within clinical teams, eg critical review, ward rounds, or discharge meetings. The contribution of individual members may be monitored.
2. Between clinicians or clinical teams. This is peer review and there will be detailed review of randomly chosen cases.
2. Within a hospital, eg prescribing practices; re-admission of schizophrenics.
4. Between units or hospitals, such as the comparison of process and outcome of similar cases in two different districts of which one might be a teaching hospital; the function of Liaison Psychiatry within different medical firms or in different hospitals.
5. Regional–this might include the management of unusual or particularly difficult cases. The example in general psychiatry given was that of investigating the management of Anorexia Nervosa.
6. National–would include Health Advisory Service, the National Development Team, Training Approval Visits and the College's ECT exercise. In Scotland, the Mental Welfare Commission has an important role in monitoring care of psychiatric patients.

Audit within the service cannot be seen in vacuum. There are three main components.

1. *Resources* include the input category of performance indicators but psychiatric resources provided within the hospital must be related to community services and specific features of the neighbourhood.

   Resources in hospital include buildings, secretarial support, computers, access to laboratories and other investigations, etc. Resources in the community would also include staff and buildings but additionally, those provided by social services, including social workers and various types of hostel accommodation, children's homes or respite provisions, those provided by education such as educational psychologists and those in the voluntary sector such as the Richmond Fellowship and the Samaritans. Demographic data concerning social class, owner-occupancy, unemployment, etc., are all relevant (Hirsch, Psychiatric Beds and Resources: Factors Influencing Bed Use and Service Planning).
2. *Process*, the second major component, comprises what is done to the patient during diagnosis and treatment. One measure of quality is the satisfaction of the patient and/or the nearest relative, and other is the personal cost born by the patient or relative in terms of pain, inconvenience and indignity.
3. *Outcome*, the third major component, presents major difficulties in psychiatry in terms of how and when it should be measured. Mortality is rarely applicable as death is an uncommon outcome except in psychiatry of old age and even there presents difficulties. Should death be rated as the worst possible outcome?

A simple rating scale of global improvement ranging from 0 = no change to 4 = complete recovery was used in the study of in-patient treatment at the Cassel hospital (Denford et al, 1983; Rosser 1988). However, since many patients have complex psychopathology, others have used multiple measures which can be conflicting where a patient is rated as improved in mood but having more problems of social impairment. As well as complex psychopathology, there is also often a problem of chronicity. A helpful idea is that of 'met needs'. Assessment of Needs, as described by Wing and his colleagues, is based on the following:

(1) Need is present when (a) a patient's functioning falls below and threatens to fall below some minimum specified level, and (b) this is due to some remedial, or potentially remediable, cause.
(2) A need (as defined above) is met when it has attracted some at least, partially effective intervention, and when no other interventions of greater effectiveness exist.
(3) A need (as defined above) is unmet when it has attracted only partially effective or no intervention and when other interventions of greater potential effectiveness exist.

Scales of disability and distress can be applied to psychiatry and to a variety of medical and surgical specialities (Rosser, 1988).

For the purposes of planning services, measures of quality of life are being developed from descriptions of states as judged by different groups. Such global indices combined with measures of prognosis form the basis of Quality Adjusted Life Years (QALY).

IV. Implementation of Audit

Clinicians will recognise from the account of clinical audit above many examples of good practice. Other methods of audit also being carried out may be improved upon such as making the review of case notes mandatory by all visiting approval teams.

Audit has an important educational function for senior doctors as well as for those more junior. It is most beneficial when all grades of medical practitioners work together.

However, unless the reviews of clinical practice as encompassed in audit lead to improvement in patient care, the collection of data is a waste of time.

Mitchell and Fowkes (1985) suggest a 'Cycle of Audit'.

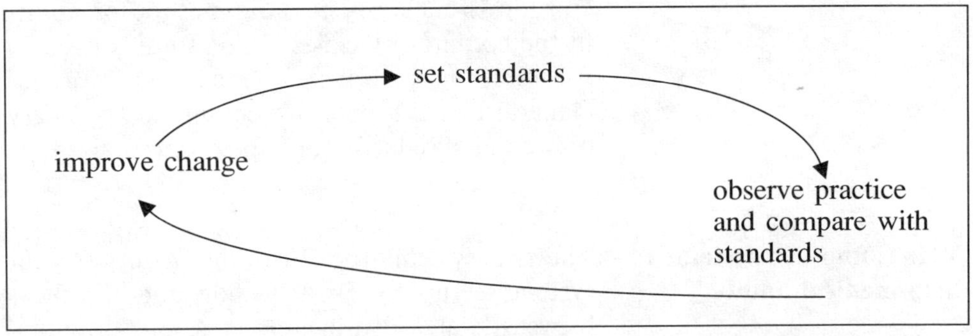

How to begin: It is a mistake to be over-ambitious. A simple project with minimum of cost in terms of both time and money expended is recommended as a start. Peer review meetings should be brief and no more than monthly to start until such time as all are able to make a regular, more substantial commitment. Other forms of audit should start by addressing only one question. A modest project successfully undertaken will generate ideas as well as increase enthusiasm.

Clinicians will find the booklet on Medical Audit by Charles Shaw, published by the King's Fund very helpful.

The Southampton psychiatrists have published a paper in the Bulletin describing how audit was put into practise in general psychiatry. (Guy Edwards, J, Nunn, C M H, and Ricketts, B S (1987)).

Confidentiality: since review of cases, especially those chosen at random can appear threatening to some, confidentiality of the doctors concerned as well as of patients should be preserved. Results of audit should be published and not suppressed or diluted for the purpose of obtaining contracts for medical services as suggested in the NHS Review White Paper.

Participation of all consultants should be encouraged and sufficient time allowed. The experience of those already involved in audit has shown that voluntary participation is effective and the benefits such that the majority of consultants are enthusiastic.

V. Management Appraisal

It is recommended that all clinicians, including psychiatrists, should take the initiative for clinical audit. It should not be imposed or prescribed by management. Measures of quality must be given at least the same emphasis as measures of quantity. Audit can and should be used for showing up deficiencies in resources as well as for improving process and outcome.

The College recommends that every consultant should be allowed to devote one session a week to audit. The College has also stated its belief in a regular multidisciplinary forum for auditing management which should complement the auditing of medical and clinical procedures.

VI. Future Development of Audit in Psychiatric Practice

The research currently under way on assessment of needs and on global indices of health are highly relevant. The work in progress of monitoring the Daily Living Programmes by Professor Marks will also provide much to guide others in auditing new or existing services.

Particular problems exist in the psychiatric specialities. As pointed out by the Working Group from the Child and Adolescent Section, family work is hard to measure and to evaluate. Community based work as in the psychiatry of Old Age and the psychiatry of Mental Handicap requires appraisal over a period of a year in the community rather than as 'consultant episodes', but no systematic method of auditing such care of chronic cases in the community exists. Pilot studies need to be established.

Simple suggestions such as the improvement of discharge letters to General Practitioners can be pursued by every consultant and offer an ideal of setting standards for junior doctors.

VII. Computer systems to help medical audit

The two systems the Working Group are considering are (i) The CRISP system set up by Dr P Rohde and (ii) the system by Ed Sein set up in Newcastle and also in Leicester.

VIII. Recommended Reading

1. Medical Audit - Hospital Handbook, King's Fund, edited by Charles Shaw.
2. Nicol, A R (1989) Performance Indicators in Child and Adolescent Psychiatry. published in the Psychiatric Bulletin, *13*, 94–97.

3. Guy Edwards, J, Nunn, C M H, and Ricketts, B S (1987) Three Years of Medical Audit in a Psychiatric Unit, Bulletin of the Royal College of Psychiatrists, *11*, 154–155.
4. Brewin, C R, Wing, J R, Mangen, S P, Brugha, T S, and MacCarthy, B (1987) Principles and practice of measuring needs in the long-term mentally ill: the MRC Needs for Care Assessment, Psychological Medicine, *17*, 971–981.
5. Medical Audit: A report of the Royal College of Physicians published in March 1989.
6. Royal College of Psychiatrists Research Committee Report from Pilot Survey on the Use of Depot Neuroleptics (not yet for publication).
7. Mitchell, M, and Foukes, F (1985) Audit reviewed: does feed-back of performance change clinical behaviour? Journal of the Royal College of Physicians, *19*, 251–4.
8. Cochrane, A L (1971) Effectiveness and efficiency: random reflection on Health Services, Nuffield Provincial Trust.
9. Section for the Psychiatry of Old Age: report of Working Group on Performance Indicators.
10. Health Service Indicators Group: A Report on Körner Indicators, December 1988.
11. Denford, T, Schachter, J, Temple N, Kind, P, and Rosser R (1983) Selection and outcome in in-patient psychotherapy. British Journal of Medical Psychology, *56*, 225–243.
12. Rosser, R (1988) A Health Index and Output Measures. In Walker S & Rosser R (Ed). Quality of Life Measurements, MTP Press.
13. Hirsch, S R Psychiatric Beds and Resources: Factors Influencing Bed Use and Service Planning, 1988, London, Gaskell.

Membership of the Working Party

Dr Ann Gath – Registrar and Convenor
Dr Fiona Caldicott – Sub-Dean
Dr James Higgins – Sub-Dean
Dr Norman Kaye – representing the Public Policy Committee
Professor John Wing – Research Director
Professor Michael Gelder – Chairman, Research Committee.

Approved by Council
June 1989

Quality and Outcome Measurement in Mental Health Services: Community Care for Schizophrenic Patients in West Lambeth

Dr David Melzer

Abstract

West Lambeth is an inner city London District with large homeless and ethnic minority populations. Details of a local service evaluation will be reported. These include clarified aims, a list of potentially effective interventions together with the design and results of a study to establish local service performance.

The objective of the study was to measure the clinical states, disabilities, social circumstances and service receipt of discharged patients with schizophrenia, and to examine targeting and co-ordination of services. A cross sectional survey of former in-patients was carried out with administered questionnaires one year after discharge.

77 of 86 patients aged 18 to 65 satisfied Research Diagnostic Criteria for schizophrenia. Subjects and carers were interviewed between November 1988 and June 1989.

Most former patients were living in unsupported accommodation, 8% had used day hospitals, 20% had seen CPNs and 22% of the unemployed had used day-care. 54% (CI: 42%–67%) of cases interviewed had current psychotic mental states at follow-up and 25% (CI: 15%–34%) were very poorly socially adjusted. Severely disabled and ill people did not receive more services.

We conclude that many former short-stay patients with schizophrenia were profoundly disabled, while care services were scarce, patchy, ill-coordinated and poorly targeted. Service targets were set and a second follow-up of the 18 most disabled patients was carried out in 1990 and will be described.

Introduction

West Lambeth Health Authority is situated in inner London and stretches from Waterloo Station in the north to part of Brixton in the south. It is the seventh most socially deprived district in the country and has large ethnic minority and homeless populations.[1] These factors are likely to increase the prevalence of schizophrenia in the resident population.

The district is actively moving residents from a large psychiatric hospital due for closure, into the community. There are, presently, no "new long-stay" facilities outside the acute bed provision, where the mean length of stay was 19.6 days during the period of the work described below. The local authority has little housing to offer and temporary accommodation for emergency rehousing is invariably to distant parts of north London and so inaccessible to Lambeth services. The setting for the work presented below was thus in no way a specially funded project but very much a routine service.

Formative Evaluation of a Local Service

The evaluation of a local service entails a number of steps which we will list and then describe in more detail below. The first step is the selection of a part of a service which is both important in public health terms and homogeneous enough for results of any study to be meaningful. Having selected such a care programme, the next step is to clarify its aims. The third step is then to identify those interventions which have been shown experimentally to be effective in achieving the desired aims. Armed with this knowledge, a survey or monitoring scheme can usually be designed to establish to what extent these potentially effective interventions are being delivered in practice and what outcomes have resulted.

Identifying poor outcomes without relating them to failing processes of care is of limited value if the purpose is to improve local services. If failing processes can be identified, targets for improvement can be set and then monitored. The process described, therefore, is more of a cycle of review and corrective effort, rather than a summary judgement of the service. Given this framework, some details of its application locally are set out below.

Very briefly, the following list of aims for the community care of patients with schizophrenia was adopted:

1. To reduce the personal suffering of patients.
2. To enhance their ability to care for themselves.
3. To enhance their social reactivity, especially their ability to behave in their own reasonable self interest.
4. To reduce the burden on others.

A review of the literature suggests that there is experimental evidence for the usefulness of at least the following types of interventions:

1. Medication, especially combined with simple social and other problem solving.[2]
2. Active follow-up and crisis intervention.[3, 4]
3. Rehabilitation, including family management interventions.[5, 6]

Studying process and outcome: an example

To evaluate the local community services, all schizophrenic in-patients discharged during a six month period were followed-up one year later. They and their carers were asked to volunteer to be interviewed on areas covering previous history, service or care input from any source and social circumstances, disabilities and clinical state. The detailed method is set out below.

Method:

All in-patients under the care of any psychiatric consultant in West Lambeth district, discharged between 1st November 1987 and 31st April 1988, aged 18 to 65 years, resident in the district or of no fixed abode at the time of their admission were included in an initial diagnostic screen of case-notes. Two hundred and sixty two sets of case-notes were located and screened, using Research Diagnostic Criteria[9] to establish a psychiatric diagnosis. 92 patients (35% of those screened) satisfied the criteria of (probable or definite) schizophrenia. These criteria exclude patients presenting with co-existing drug or alcohol abuse and select a 'core' presentation of schizophrenia.

Two patients were in the district transiently (one subsequently deported, one returning home overseas) and were excluded from the subsequent study.

Of the 90 eligible people, 8 refused all co-operation, one was untraceable and four had died. Relatives of the latter four volunteered to be interviewed, and thus follow-up information is available on 81 (90% of the cohort). Information was obtained directly from 59 cases. Where this was not possible a principal carer was interviewed, being the available carer with the most face to face contact with the case. Several of the interviewed carers proved to be staff members of various organisations rather than relatives. Interviews with former patients were carried out whenever possible in their own homes, approximately one year (mode 1.1 years) after their index discharge.

The study was approved by the West Lambeth Ethics Committee.

Information collected:

Basic demographic data and information relating to the first contact with psychiatric services and subsequent admissions were collected from case notes.

Interview schedules include the Present State Examination[7] (PSE), providing a standardised, structured psychiatric examination which was used with the 59 directly interviewed cases. The World Health Organisation's Disability Assessment Schedule (WHODAS)[8] involves assessment of the patient's capacity to perform specific social roles, for example, self care, social withdrawal or behaviour in emergencies. A 'Global' assessment summarises each patient's overall social functioning in relation to standards appropriate to their socio-economic background.

Also used was a questionnaire dealing with personal details, living situation, occupation, home activities, helpers, legal problems, medication, family history and interpersonal relations, derived from the Treatment Outcome Study Questionnaire (private communication) developed by the Colorado State Treatment Outcome Assessment programme.[9] A questionnaire developed by the Personal Social Services Research Unit at the University of Kent[10] was used to establish care receipt and its costs. Questions relating to service receipt aimed to establish what services were actually used and did not attempt to find out whether each service had or had not been offered at any time in the past.

Information about social circumstances and service receipt generally relates to the three-month period before interview, except where otherwise stated, while information on the clinical state and disabilities relates to the month before interview. All PSE and WHODAS interviews were carried out by one author (SM) and all the remainder were administered by GH.

Analysis:

PSE data were initially processed using the Catego program[7] and all data were analysed using SPSS-PC+[11]. Present State Examination diagnoses are presented in categories of definite psychotic, definite neurotic, all probable or non-specific diagnoses and those with no diagnosis.

The WHODAS Global disability ratings of 0, 1 or 2 are grouped together and labelled 'Fair', 3 is labelled 'poor', and 4 or 5 'very poor' social adjustment. For individual aspects of social dysfunction, categories presented are 'no', 'minimum' (minor dysfunctions, but persistent over the time period) and 'obvious', covering conspicuous and persistent failures to carry out social roles.

All confidence intervals (CI) and significance tests are based on 95% limits.

Results:

Demographic data and details of previous illness and type of admission are presented in Table 1 and Table 2. Most former patients were male and divided equally between ethnic majority and minority groups. Forty percent were under 30 years old (and a similar proportion (41%) had been admitted under sections of the Mental Health Act of 1983). There were no statistically significant differences between the cases and refusals (using Fisher's Exact tests) on each of these parameters.

Although many former patients had had long-standing illnesses (64% more than 5 years) the majority had never spent periods of longer than six months in mental hospitals. Almost two thirds of the group had had admissions at the start of the study of less than eight weeks.

Table 1 Demographic details of interviewed former patients and the surviving cohort at follow-up one year after discharge

	Interviewed cases (N=77)		Surviving cohort (N=86)	
	No	%	No	%
Age at discharge				
18–29	27	(35)	34	(40)
30–49	39	(51)	41	(48)
50–65	11	(14)	11	(13)
Sex				
Male	44	(57)	49	(57)
Female	33	(43)	37	(43)
Ethnicity				
Afro-Caribbean	32	(42)	38	(44)
Asian/other	8	(10)	9	(10)
White	37	(48)	39	(45)

Table 2 History of previous illness in interviewed cases

	No. of Cases	
	No.	%
Duration of illness		
0–4 Yrs	28	(36)
5–19	40	(52)
20+	9	(12)
Total	77	(100)
Longest ever hospital stay		
– 6 m	41	(69)
–12	10	(17)
–24	4	(7)
>24	4	(7)
Total	59	(100)
No. previous hospital admissions		
1	4	(7)
2– 5	32	(52)
6–10	20	(33)
11+	5	(8)
Total	61	(100)

Over half the patients had had six or more previous admissions during their illness, and readmission rates during the follow-up year were high, with half the sample being readmitted at least once.

(i) Clinical state and disabilities

At follow-up, approximately half (CI: 42% to 67%) of the fifty nine people examined (Table 3) showed persistent psychotic symptomatology at the time of testing, while only ten percent (CI: 2% to 18%) were free of all clinical symptoms.

Similarly, nearly half of the cases (Table 4) were considered socially disabled to varying degrees on global assessment, with a quarter (CI: 15% to 34%) rated as very poor social adjustment. The relationship between social adjustment and symptomatology is complex and will be reported elsewhere.

Table 3 Current clinical state one year after discharge of 52 PSE examined former patients

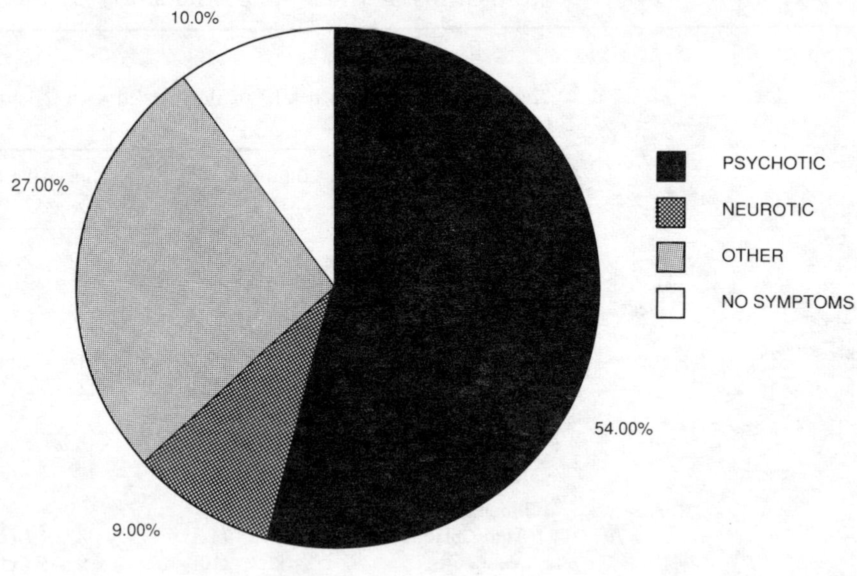

Table 4 Global Social Disability ratings one year after discharge for 77 former patients

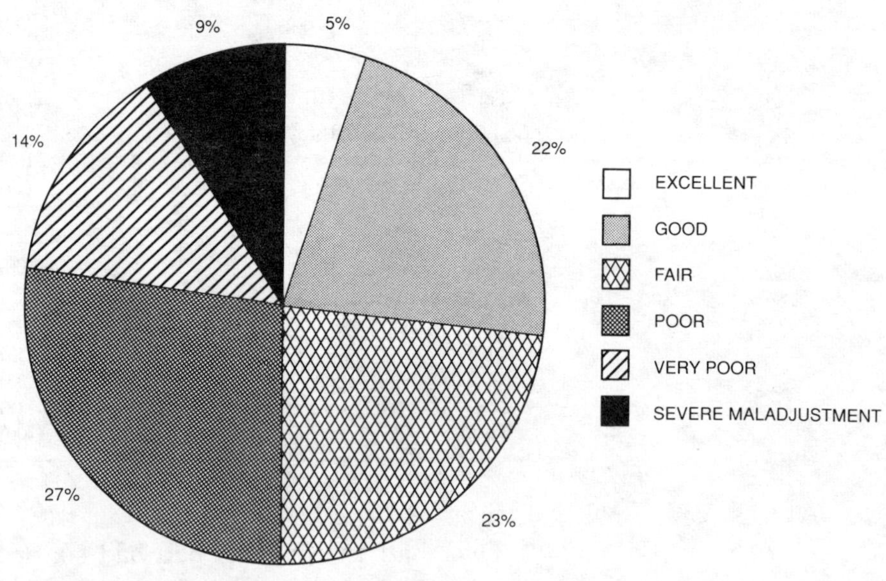

Table 5 Assessment of specific aspects of social disability one year after discharge (3 people could not be measured for outside friction)

Social dysfunction rating	Aspects of disability		
	Self care	Outside friction	Behaviour in emergencies
None	46 (60)	49 (66)	61 (79)
Minimum	17 (22)	10 (14)	3 (4)
Obvious–maximum	14 (18)	15 (20)	13 (17)

Obvious inactivity or social withdrawal were present in 40% of cases (Table 5). One in five had obvious problems resulting from a tendency to cause friction in their social contacts through, for example, inappropriate arguments, displays of anger or marked irritability. A slightly smaller number seemed obviously unable to summon help in minor crises or emergencies, including for example, sickness or accidents involving other people, or to cope with the breakdown of household equipment.

In terms of accommodation, seven people (10%) were living in temporary Bed and Breakfast or bedsit accommodation at follow-up and only 14 people were in special accommodation of any description, mostly unstaffed homes or hostels. The bulk (71%) of people were, however, living in homes of their own, including 41 (53%) in Council owned flats. In a few cases, extremely poor levels of hygiene and household maintenance were evident, sometimes combined with a lack of basic services (water, electricity, gas), cut off due to non-payment of bills.

Two former patients had slept on the streets at some time during the previous three months and four others had stayed temporarily in hostels before obtaining their present accommodation.

(ii) Informal care

Thirty five people (45%) regarded themselves as living alone (ie not sharing facilities or company) although only 22 (29%, CI 18% to 39%) actually lived in self-contained premises with no-one else. All cases had living first or second degree relatives and 51 (66%) had met with a member of their family in the previous week, although twenty two (29%, CI: 18% to 39%) had not done so for six months or more. However, only twenty five (32%) lived with or were visited at home by relatives or friends, providing direct informal care.

(iii) Employment

Only 10 (13%) of cases were working at follow-up (including part-time work) and all these were in unskilled jobs. Despite this very low employment rate, only three cases had attended industrial therapy and three had attended educational centres.

(iv) Legal difficulties

Fifteen people had had some contact with the police in the year before interview. Of these, three had been arrested, two spending one night each in a police cell, but one spent 36 nights in several different police stations before being sent to prison for one month, all on remand.

(v) Contact with services

Table 6 shows the numbers of people receiving selected medical and social services on at least one occasion in the three months prior to interview. Each of the available services, with the exception of general practice, was used by a minority of cases only, although most had used one or other medical service. It should be noted, however, that of the six not seen in medical settings, four were in the severely disabled group. The majority of the group (64%) had used some form of hospital service during the previous three months and 20% had been readmitted for inpatient stays, yet only one fifth of cases had seen a Community Psychiatric Nurse (CPN). Only 4% had used an Accident and Emergency department.

Social care services were used less than health services, the most common contact being with a social worker (30%). Few cases were in specialised accommodation of any kind and a minority used day-care facilities: 8% used social services day care, 4% voluntary and 4% private sector. For

Table 6 Percentage of the 77 former patients who were in contact with selected services during the 3 months before interview

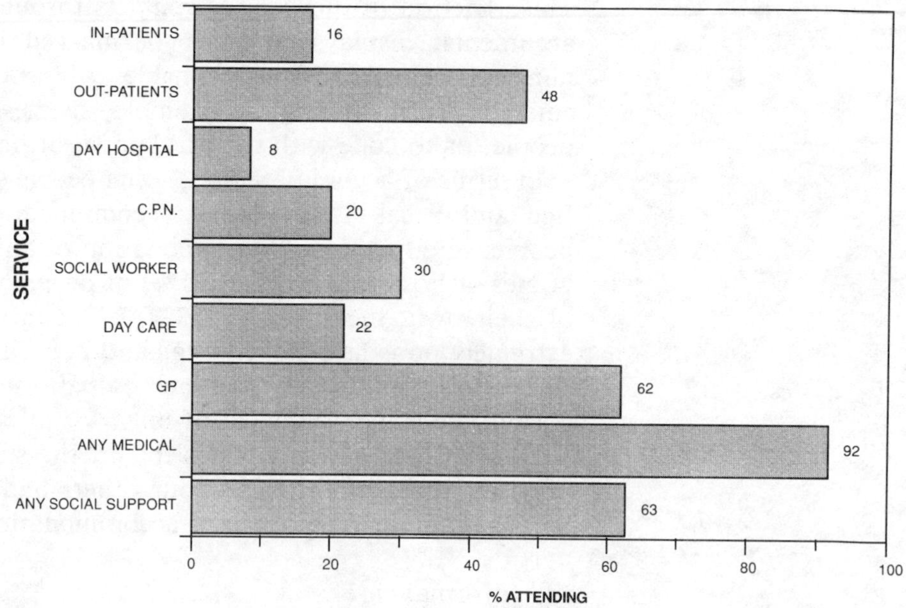

those cases receiving care, the amounts of care involved (in terms of frequency and duration of visits or average hours of attendance) varied considerably, with many of those counted as using services having in fact used them on only one of two occasions, while a very few received comparatively large amounts of care.

(vi) Equity
People who had very poor social adjustment are of special interest clearly being at most risk from neglect in the community. If care was allocated on the basis of relative need, the severely disabled group should receive more care than the rest. However, none of these former patients were in specialised accommodation or attending day hospitals and it appeared that this most disabled group received the same or fewer services, from an already low baseline, although none of the differences were statistically significant.

A well co-ordinated system of community care would use contact with one type of service to trigger the delivery of a carefully tailored package of care to vulnerable people. Lists of the care received by the 11 former patients known to have had psychotic clinical states at follow-up and who were very poorly socially adjusted were prepared. While two of these people had had no contact with any service in the previous three months, the remainder had used a haphazard combination of services, with little sign of coherent packages of care. The observation that only one of these people had seen a CPN in the previous three months is of particular concern.

Linking process and outcome

The poor performance of local services in delivering effective care needs some explanation. In operational terms, difficulties with the content and availability of clinical records was a major feature. In addition, it was rare specifically to identify patients who might need active follow-up in the community. There was no way to establish, within the service, what care was being given to any one individual. Each section within the service works independently, with its own assessment procedures and priorities: as a result, the task of organising a package of care was difficult and very time consuming.

At a policy level, management was dominated by the closure of the large mental hospital. Little attention was paid to the needs of discharged patients who are not considered, by many, to 'belong' to the service in the same way that long-stay patients do. Another difficulty was the differing views on suitable care and priorities held by different professional groups. Last, but by no means least, were the limited resources available: the absence of supported housing for revolving door patients is perhaps the most pressing need.

Setting local targets

Based on the work and analysis described above, service targets[1] were set and accepted locally. These involved, firstly, specific designation of a few of the most disabled patients. The targets were then used to ensure that the elementary social problems of this group were solved, that their medication was delivered and reviewed at least six monthly and that they were involved in some form of occupation at least twice weekly.

A second follow-up of the 18 most disabled patients from the first study was carried out a year and a half after the first follow-up, to monitor progress. Disappointingly, only marginal improvements in service contact were evident in the 14 patients who volunteered to co-operate. Disturbingly, four of these chronically disabled people, all of whom had been in contact with the services, had been arrested in the previous 6 months and two had spent time in prison in the last year.

Not infrequently, individual statistics fail to indicate the way in which certain people experience multiple neglect, sometimes because the services are simply not equipped to deal with very challenging behaviour in the community. Such people can represent service 'disasters' and the investigation of these is a powerful way of assessing process and outcome. An example is given below.

AS is a woman in her twenties who had been admitted to hospital three times in the previous twelve months. During her periods out of hospital she has lived in many different, short term forms of accommodation. On leaving hospital four months ago she found herself homeless and has had to sleep on the streets for most of the summer.

She is and has been for some time, severely disabled, with a marked tendency to violence: she has, for example, threatened people with knives (resulting in a three-week spell in prison) and is presently facing charges for assault on a child. She also, episodically, runs across busy roads, clearly risking her life.

She has been very difficult to care for in the community for some time: previous attempts to settle her in accommodation of her own have ended in failure when she has left for no apparent reason. Staffed accommodation other than hospital has not been arranged or available recently.

Not withstanding her recent admissions, her main service contacts have been with Accident and Emergency Departments and the Special Needs Housing Unit, rather than the regular community support services. Despite a previous history of schizophrenia and her homelessness, she has sometimes been refused admission to hospital on the grounds of not being psychiatrically ill at the time of presentation.

Her present situation includes having an infant in care, being homeless and having a warrant for her arrest.

Conclusion

The approach to the measurement of service quality and outcome presented above is detailed, focussed and is designed for the clear purpose of improving a service. The detail is time consuming and relatively expensive to achieve, especially as the project had to be designed from scratch.

A cheap simple approach, perhaps even a single measure, which could be produced with little effort, would be highly desirable but is difficult to imagine. Perhaps the only such measure available is to measure our own resolve to end a situation in which schizophrenia is allowed to result in hopelessness, isolation, poverty and even homelessness; to measure our determination to see the benefits of proven treatment and humane care made available to these most unfortunate people.

Acknowledgements

We would like to thank the Trustees of St Thomas' Hospital for funding this work. Many thanks are due to the former patients and relatives who volunteered to be interviewed, and the many staff members who have helped. We have received much useful advice from Dr A Lakhani, Dr T Craig, Dr P Burney, M Morgan, S Chinn and Prof L J Opit. Economic analyses have been carried out by Jenny K Beecham and Caroline Allen of the Personal Social Services Research Unit, University of Kent, Canterbury.

References

[1] West Lambeth Health Authority. Towards Informed Action For Health: First Annual Report of the Directorate of Public Health. West Lambeth Health Authority, London, 1989.

[2] Hogarty G E, et al. Drug and social therapy in the aftercare of schizophrenic patients. Arch Gen Psych 1974: 31; 603–18.

[3] Stein L I, Test M A. Alternative to Mental Hospital Treatment: conceptual model, treatment programme and clinical evaluation. Arch Gen Psych 1980: 37; 392–7.

[4] Hoult J. Community care of the acutely mentally ill. Brit J Psych 1986: 149; 137–44.

[5] Falloon I R H, Boyd J L, McGill C W, et al. Family management in the prevention of exacerbations of schizophrenia. New England Journal of Medicine: 1982: 306; 1437–40.

[6] Leff J, Kuipers L, Berkowitz R, et al. A controlled trial of social interventions in the families of schizophrenic patients: two year follow-up. Br J Psych: 1985; 146; 594–600.

[7] Wing J K, Cooper J, Sartorius N. The Measurement and Classification of Psychiatric Symptoms. Cambridge, Cambridge University Press, 1974.

[8] World Health Organisation. WHO Psychiatric Disability Assessment Schedule. Geneva, World Health Organisation, 1988.

[9] Ellis R E, Wilson N Z, Foster M F. Statewide Treatment Outcome Assessment in Colorado: The Colorado Client Assessment Record. Community Mental Health Journal 1984; 20: 72–89.

[10] Knapp M, Beecham J. Costing Mental Health Services. Psychological Medicine (in press).

[11] Norusis M J. SPSS/PC +, SPSS Inc. Chicago, 1986.

Implications for Public Health

Dr Sheila Adam

Abstract

The new public heath, heralded in the Acheson Report, is presented with a number of significant opportunities with the NHS reforms.

Health authorities (DHAs and FHSAs) are responsible for assessing the health needs of their population, determining health priorities and investing in health via the contracting process. Their achievements will be measured in health outcomes and in an improvement in health status for their resident population.

Kenneth Clarke has announced the publication of a consultation document on health targets early in the New Year. The signs so far are that this is likely to focus on the major causes of mortality such as coronary heart disease and stroke.

Whilst welcoming a move to explicit health targets, for which health authorities and managers will clearly be responsible, a number of issues arise including:

- who will determine health priorities?
- what ideology and values will be applied?
- how will the targets be influenced by the perceived availability of effective preventive or therapeutic interventions?
- how will the baseline position and subsequent progress be assessed?

Public health physicians can occupy a key role as advocates for the public health and as the interface between the community, users of the NHS, professional staff, health service managers and other relevant agencies.

The challenge for public health is to use this pivotal position to exploit the new opportunities of better health, both physical and mental.

Introduction or "would we have started from here?"

The NHS reforms which follow the publication of the three White Papers - "Promoting Better Health", "Working for Patients" and "Caring for People" - offer significant opportunities to those attempting to practice the new public health.

Few of us would have chosen to start from here and I would share the anxieties of those who discuss the potential downside of the separation of purchasing and provision, the market place and the simplistic approach to consumerism.

At the same time the organisational destabilisation which has resulted has many advantages for those who wish to achieve major change. I believe that our role is to ensure that the reforms are implemented so as to secure improvements in the health of the public. This is, of course, a ringing phrase which begs a number of questions to which I will return, but I think it provides a key organisational focus for the new public health as heralded in the Acheson Report.

April 1991 and beyond

Health authorities (DHAs and FHSAs) will be responsible for assessing the health needs of their population, determining health priorities and investing in health through the new contracting process. Their achievements will be measured in health outcomes and in an improvement in the health status of their resident population. RHAs will have a slightly more mystical role in regulation and market managing, and in monitoring the achievements of DHAs and FHSAs. My own view is that enquiry of health status should become an increasingly important theme for RHAs. This will involve some concept of equity across the range of threats to health and well-being.

The Departmental view on the key importance of health status and health outcomes has become clearer in the last four months. At a conference of health authority chairs and general managers on 17 July 1990 Duncan Nichol highlighted eight critical aspects of the NHS reforms indicating the importance which is attached to health needs assessment, health outcomes and the quality of care. This speech was also the first hint that national health targets were coming over the horizon. Kenneth Clarke, in his speech at the Conservative Party Conference, placed great emphasis on the development of health targets. He highlighted areas of concern including premature mortality and waiting lists/times. We could debate the validity of waiting lists as a ''health'' target but, nevertheless, this speech represents a real commitment to the concept. A consultation document is promised early in the new year. The shift from health care to health represents a fundamental change.

Table 1 Key strategic benefits

1. Comprehensive and systematic assessment of local health care needs.
2. Strategic planning to improve health rather than health services.
3. Balance of prevention and treatment.
4. Advances in measurement of outcome and quality.
5. Boost to evaluation of clinical practice and cost effectiveness.
6. Better integration of primary and secondary care.
7. Greater involvement of doctors and nurses in management.
8. Improved patient or consumer perspective.

Duncan Nichol, 'Working for Patients into the 90's'', 17 July 1990

Table 2 Kenneth Clarke health targets

'. . . for some of the main causes of disease and premature death'
'. . . heart disease, cancer, asthma and diabetes'
'. . . the next ten years to the year 2000'
'. . . coronary heart disease, where a possible target could be a reduction of 25% in premature deaths by 2000'
'. . . drawn from the range of NHS activity from prevention to treatment'

9 October, 1990

Whose health targets?

To return to some of the earlier begged questions. The discussion so far on health needs and health targets has hinged very much on better information and more elegant models. Given time, the problems can be solved-there is a right answer. Unfortunately, this approach tends to omit or fail to address the ideologists and values which will underpin any decisions on health targets. There is almost certainly no right answer, but a series of options.

For example, the determination of the criteria which will result in a health need becoming a health target will have a major influence on the national health priorities. The epidemiological positivists will tend to opt for one of the top categories-demonstrable problem, information more or

Table 3 Criteria to establish health targets: examples

- reduce premature mortality
- reduce preventable mortality
- reduce preventable morbidity
- increase immunisation rates
- increase uptake of screening programmes
- reduce prevalence of diseases which are heavy consumers of inpatient care
- reduce prevalence of behaviours which place people at risk of ill health
- increase quality of life as perceived by population

less available and reasonable understanding of interventions. Managers may be more interested in criteria which relate to resource consumption. Egalitarians may focus on risk factors–intervention here will address many problems of inequity. The public may be more interested in how they feel, and will not necessarily relate this to the presence or absence of definable disease. Individual professionals would promote their own particular area of expertise. Pressure groups and other advocates will argue their corner. All will advance their supporting evidence. The political response is understandably unpredictable.

This debate has not yet started despite the NHS being in its 43rd year. Arguments about priorities remain rooted in health care not in health. Undue influence is exerted by managers and professionals–this latter is particularly worrying because the power relationships within and between professional groups. Too much of the discussion is tinged with special pleading which ranges from effective advocacy to shroud-waving.

I believe that the consultation on health targets provides the hook on which to hang what must be an open and wide-ranging debate. At the same time, we must begin to work with health targets–using the debate not as a delaying tactic but as a means to improve and refine. An element of cognitive dissonance may be helpful.

The adoption of national health targets which will provide the basis for the agreement of local health targets will serve a number of purposes. Perhaps I could highlight just two–the inclusion of health improvement in the assessment of health authority and individual performance and the encouragement to DHAs and FHSAs to work more closely together.

The public health agenda

The public health agenda is a busy one–especially for a specialty which is still recovering from the horrors of the 70's and 80's. The future for public health is bright–the present tough.

I think the major task are as follows:

1. to push the development of health targets on two levels. First, to demonstrate the value of beginning to establish and hold people to account for the delivery of better health. And second, to stimulate the open and wide-ranging debate which will enable a more explicit approach to the determination of health priorities.
2. to use the strengths of the public health role which is both rooted in public health advocacy and managerially legitimate. There has been a tendency to see these two key roles as either/or. For those public health physicians who understand and enact the two components, retaining credibility within and outside the organisation, the whole is potentially far greater than the sum of the parts. The Annual Health Report is one concrete example of where advocacy and managerial influence can be effectively combined.

3. to improve the interfaces between practice and research and between practice and teaching. We are talking about a very different way of doing public health, and this must be reflected in a more effective partnership of practitioners with those in research and with those who are teaching the next generation. Many new skills are required – epidemiological, social science and managerial to name only three. The impact will go way beyond public health and should lead to a wider re-orientation of research and of pre-qualification and continuing education.
4. to begin to articulate new approaches to equity and to quality of life. Some fundamental decisions need to be made about equity not least to inform resource allocation and investment decision. We also need a better understanding of measures of quality of life so that the debate on health needs and outcomes shifts from the negative indices of mortality and morbidity to the more positive indicators of health, well-being and fulfilment.

Public health and mental health

Finally, let me turn specifically to mental health. I believe that the public health contribution in this field has been undistinguished. For reasons which I do not understand, the practice of psychiatric epidemiology and mental health services research have often been separated from parallel work relating to physical disease. For example, the London School of Hygiene which provides a home for over a hundred epidemiologists has no focus for mental health. In London psychiatric epidemiology has predominantly operated from within the psychiatric community. This may have had many advantages but the disadvantages are also apparent, with the lack of engagement of public health physicians leading to poor understanding and a failure to exploit the management role of public health.

Between the public health and mental health communities we need:

1. to ensure that mental health is included in the development of work on health needs, health outcomes and health targets.
2. to enable public health physicians to achieve a more holistic approach to mental health. Much emphasis has been placed on the problems of those people with mental illness and mental handicap who are long-stay hospital residents – presumably reflecting the focus on health care and use of resources. Public health needs to build more expertise in advising purchasers on the best "packages of care" for diagnosis, treatment and continuing care. In particular, we need to draw attention to the opportunities for preventing mental illness and mental handicap, and promoting mental health and well-being. The literature in this field is not well-known within public health, and we undoubtedly miss a number of chances within existing services to achieve improvements in these areas.
3. to ensure that an accessible information resource is established to cover, for example, mental health needs, effective intervention, investment appraisal, the roles of the NHS and other agencies and the view of users and the public. On this last point the naive simplicity of the White Paper needs to be challenged. Decades of experience, especially among social scientists, have demonstrated the complexity of obtaining valid information from either users or the wider public. Recent work in the NHS has not been encouraging with examples of failure to appreciate the difficulties in interpreting data and to take a sufficiently comprehensive approach. In particular, there has been a tendency to concentrate on patients' experiences, rather than also including their expectations and their perceptions of the outcome to their episode of care.

Conclusion

I have focused on the implications for public health of the re-orientation away from health care to health. Much could also be said about the new emphasis on quality of health care and on medical audit, but these issues have been addressed by other and more expert speakers. Suffice it to emphasise the role of public health in ensuring the implementation of medical and clinical audit and in working with clinicians to develop and meet quality standards.

I have also only mentioned in passing the importance of closer collaboration between primary and community care and hospital care, as well as between the NHS and other agencies. What I have sketched out is a challenging agenda for public health which covers the whole range of professional and managerial skills. I believe that the Acheson Report and the NHS reforms have given us an unparalled range of openings in our drive to improve the public's health.

Discussion from Workshop 2

Measurable Outcomes: their relevance to service provision

Group I

1. There should be continuous dialogue and flexibility between purchaser and provider units–this would require the specific involvement of managers, Directors of Public Health Medicine and clinicians.

2. The basis of dialogue would be to share and compliment the skills of all those involved in assessing needs and the financial and human resources required against specific diagnostic related groups. This would also take specific account of variations in mental health needs and services in local District and metropolis catchment areas who are competing with units.

3. Royal College guidelines and the criteria contained in Rachel Jenkins paper could provide District Psychiatric Units the basis from which to move forward when considering outcomes and equity of care of patients and carers.

4. An advantage of the new system could be to provide/promote country wide units for certain specialities eg anorexia–this would generate resources and provide a national service/resource to be cascaded down to District/units.

Group II: Outcomes and Purchaser

1. In the absence of information on the health of the population it was agreed to support the measurement of outcomes of health care as a proxy for the health needs of a specific area. On this basis, for purchasing authorities to have a clear idea of the state of health of the population within District boundaries, they would need to draw up a blue print of the use of services.

2. This blueprint in conjunction with considering the social deprivation factors within the District would be pre-requisites to the measurement of outcomes.

3. Standards and budgets for service outcomes would be based on detailed research evidence where available, eg the effectiveness of individual care plans; the involvement of professional colleagues in the development of care plans.

4. It is, therefore, important that clinical audit in psychiatry be included in contracts. Emphasis would also be given to the role of GP's, CHC's and consumers in monitoring the effective use of care plans. (Also see Group III A/B point 7 re suicides).

5. Secondary and tertiary prevention to be effectively monitored as appropriate through the contract process of evaluation of rehabilitation service re contact with patient and assessing long term continuing care.

Group IIIA

1. A clear definition is required for the objectives of the service which must meet the needs of prevention on both a narrow and wide remit eg prevention of the number of suicides, the drugs misuse register to the requirements for assimilating people back into the community after episodes of mental illness.

2. Services specifications must be designed to meet objectives of present service development.

3. Many outcome measures are hard to define or are related to long term issues eg child and adolescent psychiatry. Strongly need to consider systems and processes for communication to ensure:

    1. effective care plans for long term patients;
    2. successful assimilation of patients back into the community;
    3. appropriate follow-up procedures for homelessness/relapses.
    4. Contracts should reflect targets and priorities based on the measurement of outcome since service development will be defined by the health needs of the population coupled with cost effective resources.

Group IIIB

1. Audit
   This must be kept simple and have clear information requirements based on the quality of care and processes involved in measuring outcomes.

2. Outcome Measure
   Must have clear defined aims and there must be a clear system of communication to ensure and accelerate the flow of information especially clinical research. Confidentiality to be maintained as appropriate.

3. Outcome Measures
   Very important to identify who defines the outcome-the user, purchaser and provider. Strong support for user involvement ie patient and informal carer.

4. Consensus view that initially there should be minimum measurement and develop measurement systems as required by objectives arising from outcome. (also see Group IV parts 4-5)

5. Identification and targeting of priority groups must be carefully based upon local priorities as identified by needs assessment of the health of the population. Caution should be taken in case of conflict amongst interested care groups and particular consideration be given to assessing unmet need in these instances.

6. Quality of life-It is important that all systems/processes of communication take account of confidentiality, privacy and politeness-particularly so when analysing daily work with patients.

7. Need for education programme for other bodies who deal with specific high risk groups eg suicides, NB these people often visit GP before committing suicide. Function of audit to look at coroners report, referrals by who and when etc.

8. Access to non-NHS information to facilitate assessment of need, eg police convictions re alcohol.

9. Evaluation of future cost effective analysis in certain areas eg psychotherapy–the link between training and costs to future benefit of population.

Group IV

1. Specification for contracts should be practical, based on local needs, but in principle comparable between Districts.

2. Validity of information should be based on meaningful and reliable recorders such as health indicators *but also* social deprivation factors; housing and homelessness.

3. Effective use of data/research available is vital. This involves the use of guidelines for systematic monitoring of daily work. The production of a Directory which could detail feasible/affordable research instruments and guidance on where to use them would be invaluable.

4. It would be beneficial for the provider to measure the outcomes. Having identified an objective with best/worst predictions and a system to mark progress this information through a key worker or review process could be fed back into the central system and influence the planning of future activities. Clinicians voiced caution on the effect of such information on resource allocation and the independence of groups who do not wish to be monitored.

5. Imperative to establish the quality control loop (monitoring and feedback system) before directly linking outcomes to purchasing, since we must clearly identify what the outcomes are telling us–particularly regarding unmet needs in relation to service provision.

Printed in the United Kingdom for HMSO
Dd293073 6/91 C10 G443 10170